NURSING RESEARCH IN ACTION

Nursing Research in Action

Exploring, Understanding and Developing Skills

3rd Edition

Philip Burnard, Paul Morrison and Heather Gluyas

palgrave
macmillan

First edition 1990
Reprinted five times
Second edition 1994
Reprinted six times
Third Edition 2011

Published by
PALGRAVE MACMILLAN

Palgrave Macmillan in the UK is an imprint of Macmillan Publishers Limited,
registered in England, company number 785998, of Houndmills, Basingstoke,
Hampshire RG21 6XS.

Palgrave Macmillan in the US is a division of St Martin's Press LLC,
175 Fifth Avenue, New York, NY 10010.

Palgrave Macmillan is the global academic imprint of the above companies
and has companies and representatives throughout the world.

Palgrave® and Macmillan® are registered trademarks in the United States,
the United Kingdom, Europe and other countries.

ISBN: 978-0-230-23167-2

This book is printed on paper suitable for recycling and made from fully
managed and sustained forest sources. Logging, pulping and manufacturing
processes are expected to conform to the environmental regulations of the
country of origin.

A catalogue record for this book is available from the British Library.

10   9   8   7   6   5   4   3   2   1
20 19 18 17 16 15 14 13 12 11

Printed in China

To Sally, Aaron and Rebecca
and Franziska – Mo chuisle – Sarah and Maeve
and Alan – the wind beneath my wings

Brief Contents

Contents

List of Figures and Tables

Figures

Tables

Preface

This book is aimed primarily at novice researchers in different contexts. Since the publication of the first and second editions of the book there have been many changes in emphasis across the major domains of nursing – higher levels of practice acuity and changing patterns of illness, new modes of delivery in education and a much greater expectation that practice is underpinned by quality research. In addition the political climate has changed to the extent that there is a much greater awareness of the social determinants of health and wellbeing, the need for evidence in decision-making at all levels, and growing consumer expectations are placing an increasing onus on clinicians to be able to demonstrate that their practice is evidence based.

Moreover we have also been part of those changes as clinicians, educators, managers and researchers and have come to appreciate the diverse learning needs of students and practitioners when coming to terms with this fast-paced world of nursing. We are fortunate in that we (as authors) have had (collectively) a wide range of experiences in practice, managerial, educational and research settings in the United Kingdom and Australia leading to opportunities to work with, supervise and teach people with different needs.

Experienced nurses who hold senior administrative positions may have trained in an era where research was not an essential element of nursing work. More recently educated graduates may have completed a research subject at undergraduate level or had research integrated across other theoretical units within a course. In some current undergraduate programs students may complete a small project or, more rarely, undertake an honours year which is a much more rigorous training for research, but in a small and very focused area. Those undertaking postgraduate courses may be re-visiting research subjects afresh after some years in practice.

While there are many excellent books on research that can be used to learn about nursing research and research more generally albeit in a rather passive manner, this book is quite different in that we encourage you to take a much more active approach to your learning by engaging you with exercises and activities designed to challenge and support you at the same time as you explore and develop research skills. We believe as Kurt Lewin (1890–1947) so eloquently stated that 'Learning is more effective when it is an active rather than a passive process' – in other words our learning is greatly enhanced when we try things out for ourselves instead of just reading about ideas and concepts and processes.

Whatever path you have trodden to date it is likely that your skill base in research may be a bit 'thin' and needs extending and expanding given the context described above. We are using the term 'novice researcher' to refer to those nurses who need to extend their skills and understanding of research as a prerequisite for contemporary nursing practice.

How to use this book

The book may be used in a variety of ways:

- It may be used on its own as a learning package. A nurse working through the book on his/her own can do the various exercises and follow up the diverse approaches through reference to the many books and articles recommended throughout the text. S(he) may also do further reading via the suggested reading lists contained in each chapter. However learning about research in a student group where active participation and engagement with the ideas are encouraged is more likely to result in deep learning, which promotes understanding and application in a wider context.

- The book may also be used as part of a student-centred learning programme. Nurse educators and lecturers are realizing, increasingly, that people learn at different speeds and that their learning needs vary. Thus, the book can be tailored to suit the varying needs of the people using it. For some, it will help to work right through the book as an introduction to the research process in nursing. For others, it will be more appropriate to select certain chapters relating to specific skills.

- It may be used as a programme of guided reading. The book unfolds logically to cover all the stages of the research process. As it does this, a wide and varied range of references is offered. Readers are given the opportunity to sample different sorts of research. Thus the book can be a rich source of reference for the person who wishes to become familiar with a broad view of the research literature. Examples of research projects are drawn not only from nursing but from the whole range of social sciences. We feel that it is important that nurses sample and explore all sorts of approaches to doing research.

■ The book may be used as a resource. Many of the passages can serve as the means by which ideas are sparked off or the next stage of a research project is planned. The references offered throughout the book will also be useful in gaining new leads and developing thoughts and plans. While some students may benefit from working through the book in a more structured classroom format, those with some research experience may find it helpful to dip into areas of the book as a cookbook to be explored in a more unstructured way.

■ Experiential learning, or learning directly through personal experience, is also a growing trend in nurse education. The book is not only theoretical in nature. It invites the reader to complete a range of exercises to reinforce learning. Thus, used in a group context and with group reflection after the completion of each exercise, the book can be used as an aid to facilitating experiential learning. If the book is used in this way, it is recommended that the following issues are borne in mind:

  ■ The lecturer or facilitator should appreciate that each student will tend to find different results at the end of each exercise. It is useful if the lecturer does not try to force a particular point of view on the group but allows for these differences of perception.

  ■ Plenty of time should be allowed for the completion of the exercises and about an hour should be allowed afterwards for discussion or 'processing' of the activity so that the full range of learning can be identified and shared across the group.

Preparing for activities

We use lots of activities and exercises in this book to help you to learn. In some cases you may be completing these alone or with a small group as part of a course. In other instances you may be teaching yourself about research in order to undertake a small study at work. Whatever your particular circumstances we assume that you have access to a nursing focused learning resource centre which will provide access to databases, the internet, books and journals in hard copy. You will also need a notebook and pen or a computer with access to the internet. One of the most critical things you will need is time – and you will need to build in reading time into your schedule to ensure that learning is optimized. And when you read things you must make good notes as you go and file these in a disciplined and systematic manner. These resources are essential to complete the exercises successfully.

Evaluating the activities

As you complete each of the activities it will be useful if you note down: what you learned in the exercise; how you can use what you learnt; and, what you need to learn next. If you are working in a group, discuss your evaluation with others in the group. You may want to use what others have noted to add to your own evaluation. It is really important to make these notes as you go as the activity of writing will help with understanding and on occasion raise new questions for you to follow up.

The term 'supervisor'

People engaged in research usually love talking about their work – the good times and the bad times. However people who do research usually *need* someone to talk to. Talking about your research with other people will help you to think in a clear and critical fashion. It will encourage reflection. Whether you are a student completing a project as part of your course work, a Masters, or PhD student or a clinician engaged in evaluating the evidence for best practice, you will need someone to talk about your research work.

As a student you may be assigned an advisor, mentor, a critical friend or tutor to help. In the university context these people are usually called supervisors. As a clinician you may be part of a small research team that is led by one or two people sometimes from other disciplines. Whatever your particular circumstances, if you are doing research having someone to talk with is essential. You may be surprised to know that even experienced researchers talk to other people about their work – asking for advice about analysis or suggestions about particular issues in sampling or practical problem solving.

In this book we will use the term 'supervisor' to cover the range of people you may call on for help along your own journey of learning about research. The word supervisor will not fit easily with everyone but it probably captures the experiences of many readers, especially if we think of a supervisor as a person who helps with planning, problem solving, debriefing, methodology and critical thinking. In addition, you can have more than one supervisor – it is a good idea to talk to several people. Using this single term will also help to enhance the readability of the book.

Your personal library

As you learn more and more about research you will find it helpful to build up a small library of textbooks that you constantly refer to. You will be surprised how useful these will be over the years. Here are some of the books (below) we refer to constantly throughout this book. They are all very well written and easy to read; they are packed with high quality information that is easy to understand and they are engaging and affordable. You will no doubt find others to add to your personal library that are particularly appealing to you.

SUGGESTED READING

Bell, J. (2005) *Doing Your Research Project: A Guide for First-time Researchers in Education and Social Science* (4th edn). Milton Keynes: Open University Press.

Gerrish, K. & Lacey, A. (eds) (2006) *The Research Process in Nursing* (5th edn). Oxford: Blackwell Publishing.

Newell, R. & Burnard, P. (2010) *Vital Notes for Nurses: Research for Evidence-Based Practice* (2nd edn). Oxford: Blackwell Publishing.

Robson, C. (2007) *How to Do Research Project: A Guide for Undergraduate Students.* Oxford: Blackwell Publishing.

It may seem somewhat daunting when we ask you to read some of these at first but our intention is not that you read these through from cover to cover straightaway. Instead we offer these because we know you can dive into different sections of these as novice researchers and extend your learning around the particular activity or exercise we focus on.

The journey begins

The book offers an exploratory approach to most aspects of the research cycle. Both quantitative and qualitative methods of doing research are addressed as are a variety of ways of collecting and analysing data. The reader is encouraged to draw up a research proposal, identify proposed data collection methods and methods of analysis and is then directed towards writing up the project. A series of guideposts and specific readings is offered throughout the text to illuminate certain aspects of the topics under discussion. Overall, the book should serve as a practical introduction to the business of doing and thinking critically about research in nursing.

We have been unable to find a satisfactory solution to the problem of non-sexist language. Using 'they' as both singular and plural was considered but deemed to be clumsy. In the end, we settled for the nurse as 'she', though we wish to acknowledge that the reader may just as easily read 'he' in its place. The issue of how to write clear and unambiguous non-sexist prose remains a challenge both for the writer generally and for the person who is reporting research.

More than anything else, we hope that the book will help you to think critically about the issues involved in doing research. It is important to learn not to tacitly accept information and facts, as students often do to pass examinations, but to question the assumptions, research findings and methodological issues underpinning these. Indeed this questioning attitude should be a core element in your professional practice whether or not you do your own research.

PHILIP BURNARD
PAUL MORRISON
HEATHER GLUYAS
2011

Acknowledgements

The authors would like to thank Bunny le Roux, formerly Principal Lecturer, Department of Applied Statistics and Operational Research, Sheffield Hallam University for permission to reproduce the statistical exercise in Chapter 8. We would also like to thank Pat Tandy, Academic Planning Librarian from the library at the University of Canberra for assistance and advice.

The authors and publishers would also like to thank Thomson Reuters for granting permission to reproduce Figure 3.3: a screenshot of EndNote® © Copyright 2011 Thomson Reuters.

Every effort has been made to trace all the copyright holders, but if any have been inadvertently overlooked the publishers will be pleased to make the necessary arrangement at the first opportunity.

About the Authors

Philip Burnard

Philip is Emeritus Professor of Nursing at Cardiff University, Wales, UK. He is the author of many books and papers and has taught internationally. His research interests have included interpersonal skills and counselling, stress and culture in nursing. He continues to work with colleges and universities around the world.

Paul Morrison

Paul is Professor of Nursing and Health Studies and Dean of the School of Nursing and Midwifery at Murdoch University in Western Australia. He has a long-standing interest in the mental health area and the education of health professionals. A major focus of his research over the years has been the evaluation of services for consumers. More recently he has published a number of papers in the area of health promotion. Paul also works as a psychologist in private practice. He is a Chartered Psychologist and an Associate Fellow of the British Psychological Society.

Heather Gluyas

Heather is Associate Professor in Nursing at Murdoch University School of Nursing & Midwifery in Western Australia and Adjunct Associate Professor in the School of Nursing at University of Notre Dame. She has had a varied career in nursing with a strong clinical background in Critical Care and Aged Care. She joined academia six years ago to pursue her interest in patient safety and completed doctoral studies in clinical governance. Heather has presented widely in Australia and internationally in the areas of clinical governance and professional issues in nursing.

1

An Overview of the Research Process

- To identify definitions of research;

- To identify examples of different sorts of research;

- To outline the stages of the research process;

- To help you plan your research project in a structured and methodical way.

Introduction

Many people are put off by the word 'research'. Yet the word is everywhere these days and it is unlikely to disappear from our professional vocabulary any time soon. Seasoned health professionals, aspiring practitioners and first year students of nursing commonly report that the word 'research' elicits thoughts of 'dreadfully hard statistics', 'weird concepts', 'questionnaires', 'surveys' and 'very clever people'. Research in practice entails much more than this and you may be surprised to know that most of us are engaged in research activity everyday. Let us take the example of shopping for a bottle of shampoo.

Let us assume that most readers will share this experience or have done so in the past before shaved head fashions or baldness set in. To begin with you might describe your own hair in a particular way – as dry, greasy or normal (whatever that means). Many of the shampoo companies package their products in this way. So you set out to examine the shelves for the shampoo type that matches your particular hair. You might be a little worried about recurring dandruff so you have to take this into account too. If not, that makes your search easier. Alternatively, if you are concerned about whether the brands have been tested on animals is another factor that will influence your search. In short you are taking a position on shampoo and being clear about the things that you give value to.

As you explore the supermarket aisle where the shampoo is located you are confronted with an array of aromas and colourful bottles, pictures of shiny hair, shampoo types, different price ranges (per 100 ml), different brand names and claims about the quality and the outcomes associated with particular shampoos. Sometimes these claims are linked to studies which demonstrate how good the shampoo is and how many people are satisfied with it. Before you get to the supermarket you have been informed (primed) through TV or magazines that some shampoos will make you and your hair look beautiful and attractive. You have to make a choice now and you do. You select a shampoo brand that fits with your available cash at this point in the pay cycle, convinced that you got a bargain that will help to make you beautiful.

But it does not end there. After you have tried this shampoo for a week or two you notice that it smells great but that it does not help with the dandruff problem so you decide that you will not buy this product again. The next time you go shopping for shampoo you try something else.

While searching for shampoo you are doing research. It involves being clear about your own values and seeking out information that is useful for you. It is about observing and selecting from an array of possible factors or variables that seek our attention. It entails weighing up the claims, the evidence and the potential costs and benefits of making choices. Finally shampoo shopping, like research, often involves evaluating those choices and deciding on a new course of action to get a better outcome.

The difference between shampoo shopping and research though is that you will more than likely have a fairly clear understanding of how to evaluate and undertake your search for the right shampoo. To evaluate or undertake nursing research you will probably need to develop a clearer understanding of the processes involved.

Research has been defined in various ways. In this chapter you will be exploring some research definitions. What is more important, however, is that you will learn that almost all research goes through certain stages. If you have an understanding of these stages, it will help you in several ways. First, to read research reports and make sense of them; second, it will give you skills to critically analyse research reports; and third, if relevant you will be able to apply what you read to your own nursing environment.

In addition, a good understanding of the research process as a nurse researcher will provide a framework for you to undertake your own research projects. If you can develop the skill of breaking down your project into manageable chunks you will find it that much easier to control and to do. The first part of the chapter invites you to think about what research is; the second part offers you a format for identifying the stages that go to make up the research process. If you begin with structure, your task will be easier and thinking clearer.

The point of all this should be to enable you to *read* research reports and make more sense of them. Also, you should be able to *apply* what you read to your own working environment and to the clinical situation. You should be able to use this level of understanding to evaluate, critically, other people's research reports and evaluate their relevance (or lack of it) to the nursing environment. In the words of the social psychologist and researcher, Kurt Lewin: 'Research that produces nothing but books will not suffice' (Lewin 1946, p. 35).

SUGGESTED READING THAT WILL PROVIDE YOU WITH AN INTRODUCTION TO NURSING RESEARCH

Bell, J. (2005) *Doing Your Research Project: A Guide for First-Time Researchers in Education and Social Science* (4th edn). Milton Keynes, Oxford University Press, pp. 1–28.

Gerrish, K. & Lacey, A. (eds) (2006) *The Research Process in Nursing*, (5th edn). Oxford: Blackwell, pp. 1–15.

Godshall, M. (2010) *Fast Facts for Evidence Based Practice: Implementing EBP in a Nutshell.* New York: Springer Publishers, pp. 43–64.

Robson, C. (2007) *How to Do a Research Project: A Guide for Undergraduate Students.* Oxford: Blackwell Publishing, pp. 5–46.

Winsett, R. P. & Cashion, A. K. (2007) The nursing research process. *Nephrology Nursing Journal*, 34(6), 635–43.

Definitions of research

By the end of this section you will have discovered:

- How to define research;
- The meanings or usage of certain words.

Some definitions of research

Research has been defined as:

> The systematic study of materials and sources in order to establish facts and reach new conclusions.
>
> (Compact Oxford English Dictionary 2005, 3rd edn)

Here are some more definitions:

> The major rationale for conducting research is to build a body of nursing knowledge for the improvement of patient outcomes. This is accomplished by using results of research in the provision of nursing care that is based on scientific data rather than on a hunch, gut feeling, or the way I was taught. As a profession, nursing must be accountable for providing safe, cost-effective, and efficient care.
>
> (Boswell & Cannon 2007)

> Nursing research is the systematic gathering of information to gain, expand, or validate knowledge about health and responses to health problems. Evidence-based nursing uses research-based evidence to plan and implement quality care.
>
> (Macnee & McCabe 2008)

> Research is the systematic process of collecting and analysing information (data) in order to increase our understanding of the phenomenon about which we are concerned or interested. People often use a systematic approach when they collect or interpret information to solve the small problems of daily living. Here, however, we focus on *formal research*: research in which we intentionally set out to enhance our understanding of a phenomenon and expect to communicate what we discover to the larger scientific community.
>
> (Leedy & Ormrod 2001)

> Research is a process of gathering data in a strictly organised manner...Research is a process of testing a stated idea or assertion (the hypothesis) to see if the evidence supports it or not...Research is a process of engaging in planned or unplanned interactions with or interventions in parts of the real world, and reporting on what happens and what they seem to mean.
>
> (Davies 2007)

=========================== **EXERCISE 1.1** ===========================

Aim of the exercise: To explore some definitions of research.

What to do: Read the above definitions and consider the following questions

- In what way do these definitions disagree or agree with each other?

- What is meant by the word 'scientific' in any of the definitions?

- Can you be scientific about people?

- What relationship has research to evidence-based nursing practice?

- Which definition do you prefer and why?

- Does the dictionary definition seem any different to the others? If so, what are the problems of using a dictionary to define words with specific meanings in a particular discipline?

Read through the following research reports and then consider in what ways those pieces of research support the definitions offered above. If they do not, in what ways are the above definitions inadequate, if these reports are still to be called research?

SUGGESTED READING

Goldsmith, L., Skirton, H., & Webb, C. (2008) Informed consent to health-care interventions in people with learning disabilities – an integrative review. *Journal of Advanced Nursing*, 64(6), 549–63.

Edvardsson, D. (2009) Balancing between being a person and being a patient – a qualitative study of wearing patient clothing. *International Journal of Nursing Studies*, 46, 4–11.

Day, J., Higgins, I., & Koch, T. (2009) The process of practice redesign in delirium care for hospitalised older people: a participatory action research study. *International Journal of Nursing Studies*, 13–22.

Evaluation: Discuss your conclusions with colleagues or with your supervisor. Can research be defined easily? What are the problems with definition in this field? Have your views about research changed as a result of reading research reports?

Examples of nursing research

By the end of this section you will have discovered:

- What types of research is being done in nursing;

- The connections that can be formed between nursing and other disciplines;

- The wide range of issues that have been addressed by nursing researchers.

Where do you find research reports?

Research is written up in a variety of books, articles and papers. The following list offers some sources of research material:

■ Books

■ Magazines and journals such as *Nursing Times* (Short Reports and Occasional Papers sections), *Journal of Advanced Nursing, Nurse Education Today, Nursing,* the add-on journal, *International Journal of Nursing Studies.* If you have a particular interest it is possible that there may be a specific journal that deals with this. You can use your internet search engine to search for a 'list of nursing journals'. You will turn up hundreds which deal with different aspects of nursing

■ Newspapers

■ Academic theses and dissertations –. Example weblinks: http://adt. caul.edu.au/ and http://library.open.ac.uk/find/thesis/

■ Authors and researchers

■ Remember that the inter-library loan system, available through most libraries, can arrange for you to see copies of research reports that are not available to you locally. Ask your librarian how this system works and how you can use it. Some universities now share resources with other university libraries.

■ Internet searches through the library where the library has purchased access to specific research databases or databases where the access is open.

■ Google scholar – http://scholar.google.com.au/

■ www.ncbi.nlm.nih.gov/sites/entrez (access to selected free articles from peer-reviewed journals)

■ http://dlthede.net/Informatics/Chap11InternetSearching/ OnlineJournals.html (summary of free online journal content type and availability)

■ http://www.joannabriggs.edu.au/pubs/best_practice.php

━━━━━━━━━━━━━━━ **EXERCISE 1.2** ━━━━━━━━━━━━━━━

Aim of the exercise: To explore the range of research that has been done in nursing.

What to do: Read a selection of abstracts (summaries), contents lists or papers from the following journals to discover some of the types of research that have been done in these areas:
http://www.appliednursingresearch.org/

http://emergencynurse.rcnpublishing.co.uk/
http://www.journalofadvancednursing.com/
http://www.sciencedirect.com/science/journal/13551841
http://www.britishjournalofmidwifery.com/
http://ebn.bmj.com/content/by/year

Read the section on 'Types of nursing research' to consider the range of approaches to nursing research.

Locate the *Journal of Advanced Nursing* using your library's database search engine (see Exercise 3.1 if you need guidance on how to do this). Look through this and make a note of some of the research studies that may relate to your own field of interest. It may be helpful to look through the index in the final edition for several years with a list of key words for your chosen area. Then note down one or two titles of research projects that are very different to your own areas of interest. Download and read copies of these reports. Consider the following points:

- In what way do the various research reports differ from each other?

- To what extent are the reports related to clinical nursing?

- Were the reports easy to read? Were there difficulties with any of the following:

    - the terminology used? - reading tables and statistical reports? - the author's style of writing?

- What sort of structure did the reports have? Were they clearly laid out with a series of headings and subheadings?

Evaluation: Discuss your findings with colleagues or with your supervisor. Try to discover if there is a standard format for the layout of research reports. Consider, too, the wide range of:

- nursing research topics

- approaches to research

- ways of doing research

- readability in nursing research reports. Remember: anyone who has anything important to say will not risk being misunderstood. Has this been true in your experience?

Types of nursing research

Some research projects are general and broad in approach: they study the broad canvas of nursing. Others look at a particular aspect of nursing, for example, medical nursing. Others consider one topic in nursing, for example, pain. Others, still, look only at one specific case or situation. In Figure 1.1, you can see the progression from the general to the

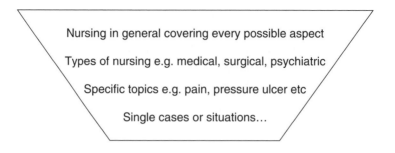

Nursing in general covering every possible aspect

Types of nursing e.g. medical, surgical, psychiatric

Specific topics e.g. pain, pressure ulcer etc

Single cases or situations...

Figure 1.1 Refining research topics from the general to the specific

specific. What will your project be: 'broad' in nature or in-depth and very specific?

Another way of considering types of research is to think about the theoretical framework adopted by the researcher. For example, some researchers study their topic from a psychological point of view, some from a sociological standpoint and others from a biological position. If you wanted to research the topic of pressure ulcers, there are various frameworks that you could adopt depending on what aspect of pressure ulcers you wanted to study. You may look at the psychological effects on patients who need to have regular and painful dressings done to care for their pressure ulcers; or you may want to find if there is a relationship between the sociological situation of the person and the development of pressure ulcers; or you may be looking from a biological perspective trying to identify if the different types of dressings effect the wound healing. You might even want to look at several different aspects and combine the various approaches. In recent years, the nursing profession has begun to develop its own body of theories and models. Research is being done to clarify and validate that theoretical base.

Researchers may adopt a particular emphasis in their studies and/or build on theoretical ideas already published. Sometimes, when we begin to explore an area, we find that it comes with a readymade orientation. For example, much of the literature on pressure ulcers has a biological emphasis. So it is important to remember, when setting out to examine an area such as pressure ulcers, that you should look outside the boundaries of your professional discipline and explore how other disciplines have studied a specific issue or problem.

Stages of the research process

By the end of this section you will have discovered:

■ How to divide up the task of doing research into manageable chunks.

- How to think systematically about your research.

- How most research, irrespective of the approach that is taken, is *structured*.

- How understanding the systematic research process can help you to read research reports critically.

EXERCISE 1.3

Aim of the exercise: To identify the stages of the research process.

What to do: Find one nursing research report from two or three of the following journals (check Exercise 3.1 if you need guidance on how to access these journals through the library database). Note, when you find them, differences in style, content, layout and readability in each of the journals:

- *Nurse Education Today*

- *Journal of Advanced Nursing*

- *British Journal of Nursing*

- *Nursing Research*

- *Journal of Clinical Nursing*

- *International Journal of Mental Health Nursing*

- *International Journal of Nursing Practice*.

All of these journals use headings and subheadings in the layout of their research reports and articles.

Jot down the headings used in a nursing research report from each of the above journals and notice to what degree there are similarities and differences between the sorts of headings and subheadings used. Out of this information, try to devise a system of stages that may help to guide you through the process of doing research. Then read the guidelines laid out in the section below. To what degree do your headings coincide with ours?

Evaluation: Notice the similarity between the headings used in a written report and the stages of the research process identified below. You can use the headings that you have derived or the headings list of suggested stages in the research process below:

- to guide you in the critical evaluation of research reports

- to guide you in your planning

- to help you organize the writing up of your project.

Stages in the research process

One of the first tasks the researcher has to consider is the *structure* of his or her research work. In order to facilitate this, it is useful to write out a research proposal which is a plan of action describing specifically how you will go about each stage in the research process to complete the research project. The details of such a proposal are discussed later in this book. At the moment, it is important to focus on the broad stages of the research process and these can be enumerated as follows:

1. Deciding on the research question

2. Locating and searching relevant literature

3. Planning the project and preparing a proposal

4. Considering ethical issues and getting permission to do the research

5. Negotiating access to the research site

6. Selecting an appropriate method

7. Collecting and storing data

8. Analysing and interpreting data

9. Drawing conclusions and making recommendations

10. Writing up and presenting the findings.

This is *one* way of planning your research. You may find other outlines. The important thing is that you *plan*. Research is never a tidy process. You will often find that the stages in the research process overlap in various ways and that you will return to certain stages again and again. Despite this, it is still important to have a very clear initial plan that can serve as a template for your work.

SUGGESTED FURTHER READING ABOUT THE PROCESS OF RESEARCH

Gerrish, K. & Lacey, A. (eds) (2006) *The Research Process in Nursing* (5th edn). Oxford: Blackwell Publishing, pp. 16–30.

Newell, R. & Burnard, P. (2010b) *Vital Notes for Nurses: Research for Evidence-Based Practice* (2nd edn). Oxford: Blackwell Publishing, pp. 3–20.

Robson, C. (2007) *How to Do a Research Project: A Guide for Undergraduate Students*. Oxford: Blackwell Publishing, pp. 47–69.

Planning a research project

By the end of this section you will have discovered:

■ How to bring structure to your own project and how to plan your work. You may or may not be actually going to undertake a research project at this stage, but in developing a research proposal your understanding of the process of research will be strengthened. Each of the stages in the exercise below is described in greater detail in the following chapters.

═══════════════════ **EXERCISE 1.4** ═══════════════════

Aim of the exercise: To identify your particular learning needs in relation to developing a research proposal.

What to do: Make notes about your own research topic under the following headings. In particular note those areas which you were not sure in order to follow this up in the following chapters.

1. Deciding on the research question (this is explored in greater depth in chapter 2)

   ■ What is the general area that you are interested in?

   ■ Write a list of specific questions that you want to know more about in this area.

   ■ From this list identify the particular question that is your highest priority.

   ■ Can you write *one sentence* that sums up what you want to do?

This stage of your work is critical. If you can clarify exactly what it is that you want to research, then the other processes that follow will be that much easier. It is worth investing considerable time in undertaking the clarification of your research question. Discuss this at some length with both your supervisor and, if you are able, with other people who have had research experience. As you read more and refer to other sources of literature you may want to refine further, your research question. A good research question takes time to refine so make sure you allow yourself sufficient time to do this.

2. Locating and searching relevant literature (this is explored in greater depth in chapter 3)

   ■ Where will you go to find relevant literature?

   ■ Do you know how to use bibliographies and indexes at your library?

- What search engines are available for you to use?

- Will you have access to bibliographic software such as EndNote® (http://www.endnote.com/) or Refworks (http://www.refworks.com/) to manage the literature?

- Are you familiar with the inter-library loan system?

3. Planning the project and preparing a proposal (this is explored in greater depth in chapters 2 and 9)

   - Are there specific proposal guidelines and forms issued by your school of nursing, college or local authority?

   - Have you got someone to advise you and/or oversee your project: a supervisor?

   - Have you seen other people's proposals? If not, have a look at one soon.

4. Considering ethical issues and getting permission to do the research (this is explored in greater depth in chapter 2)

   - Will you be talking to patients, family members, members of the public or professional colleagues? If so, you will probably be required to submit your proposal to a human ethics committee. The issue of whether a research proposal should be subject to the approval of an ethics committee varies from area to area. You need to check with your own health authority or department whether your project will require ethical approval. This is a critical aspect of your work. You cannot proceed without ethical clearance if your area or department requires it.

   - An ethics committee will review your proposal carefully to weight up the risk and benefits of the planned study. Your proposal must clarify how potential risks to participants are balanced against the potential benefits of the study. It is always a good idea to talk to a member of your local ethics committee beforehand and refer to appropriate websites where the core principles that guide committee decisions are to be found, for example: http://www.nhmrc.gov.au/health_ethics/hrecs/index.htm.

   - Do you know how to make a submission to your ethics committee?

5. Negotiating access to the research site

   - Whom do you approach to get permission to meet the people you want to talk to in your research? It is usual to adopt a 'top down' approach and ask the most senior person first. You MUST ask permission to interview or talk to people. You cannot assume that no one will mind if you do not bother. Discuss the best way to manage this with your supervisor.

6. Selecting an appropriate method (this is explored in greater depth in chapters 4 and 5)

   ■ What methods have been used in this field before?

   ■ Have they been used successfully?

   ■ Is it time for a fresh approach?

   ■ What other approaches are available?

7. Collecting and storing data (this is explored in greater depth in chapters 6 and 7)

   ■ What practical considerations do you need to make with regard to collecting data? Consider, for example, the following issues:

      ■ allocation of time; - finding a place to talk to people; - expenses to cover postage, travel, typewriting/word processing;

      ■ facilities for storing data: files, paper, computer software.

8. Analysing and interpreting data (this is explored in greater depth in chapter 8)

   ■ Are you familiar with *how* to analyse data? This will be discussed in a later chapter but you must have decided how to analyse data before you begin to collect it.

9. Drawing conclusions and making recommendations (this is explored in greater depth in chapters 9 and 10)

   ■ What sort of conclusions do you anticipate drawing? If you can answer this too readily, then you are not remaining open-minded. You are tending to pre-judge the outcome of your research.

   ■ Who will be interested in your research? For what audience will you be writing?

10. Writing up and presenting the findings (this is explored in greater depth in chapter 10)

    ■ Can you type and/or use a word processor?

    ■ Have you got access to a word processor?

    ■ If not, can you afford to have your work typed by someone else?

    ■ Will you need to send copies of your report to other people?

    ■ If so, is there a standard format for such a report?

Evaluation: Talk these issues through with colleagues and with your supervisor. Note the learning needs that may have arisen as a result of doing this exercise and keep a note of them. The following chapters will help you to become proficient in undertaking the tasks alluded to in the above questions. At a later stage in your work, you may want to return and do this exercise again. Your needs, wants and skills will change as you get on with doing your research.

CONCLUSION

This chapter provides an overview of some of the critical elements in the research process as a foundation for the development of a research plan. Planning and structuring your project before you start to collect data will pay huge dividends and is a necessity. The more you are able to organize your work, the clearer you will be about the tasks you have to do. It is helpful to sit down with a large pad of paper and make a series of headings and subheadings, thus dividing up your project into smaller and smaller tasks. This process (which is sometimes known as 'outlining') can also be done on a personal computer or word processor. We strongly recommend that you convert you notes into computerized files.

Research is an ongoing process involving many drafts, steps and stages so it is a good idea to keep track of these in a methodical manner. There are some specialist software packages that may be helpful for things like concept mapping, outlining and project planning and some of these may be available freely on the internet or bundled with office software that you already have. If you want to explore these software options further then use a search engine such as Google to look for more information about them.

It is very hard to draw up a plan of research, and usually you will have to do a variety of *drafts*: not many people get it right the first time. The plan must also be *realistic*. It is easy to think of the sort of project you would *like* to do, but often it is a question of what you *can* do. Many initial plans are overambitious. Work closely with your supervisor to keep your project realistic and manageable.

The great advantage of planning your work properly in advance is that such planning nearly always leads to a much better outcome. Your research report will benefit from the planning that you put into place at the beginning of your study.

CHAPTER

Planning Your Research Project

Introduction

In this chapter we explore the process of planning the research project. In the first chapter we talked about the research proposal: your statement of intent with regard to your research. In this chapter we show you how to write one. Some of the information you need to complete a research proposal is covered in later chapters of this book. We suggest that you undertake the exercises here, now: later, and in the light of your new knowledge, you should return to this chapter and be prepared to modify your proposal.

SUGGESTED READING FOR THIS CHAPTER

Bell, J. (2005) *Doing Your Research Project: A Guide for First-Time Researchers in Education and Social Science* (4th edn). Milton Keynes: Open University Press, pp. 28–42.

Davies, M. B. (2007) *Doing a Successful Research Project: Using Qualitative or Quantitative Methods*. Basingstoke: Palgrave Macmillan, pp. 1–50.

Clarifying research problems and questions

By the end of this section you will have discovered:

- How to be clear about what your research is about.

- How other people have clarified their research problems.

- How important all this is in reading and evaluating research reports.

EXERCISE 2.1

Aim of the exercise: To identify a clear and specific research problem or question.

What to do: For this exercise, you will be encouraged to use the process known as 'brainstorming'. It is a technique that will be useful in a variety of ways throughout your research work.

Brainstorming

This is a method of generating ideas, topics and issues that can later be clarified to form a cohesive plan. You will find the technique useful in at least the following situations:

- For clarifying a research question;

- For exploring potential research methods;

- For identifying possible constraints and solutions;

- For identifying new ideas for new projects;

- For problem-solving;

- For helping to identify material for an essay or project;

- For uncovering material for a teaching session;

- For sharing a wide range of ideas in a group setting;

- For developing creativity and intuition.

Figure 2.1 shows how the brainstorming technique was used to explore thinking about how to take blood pressure (BP). Now you can

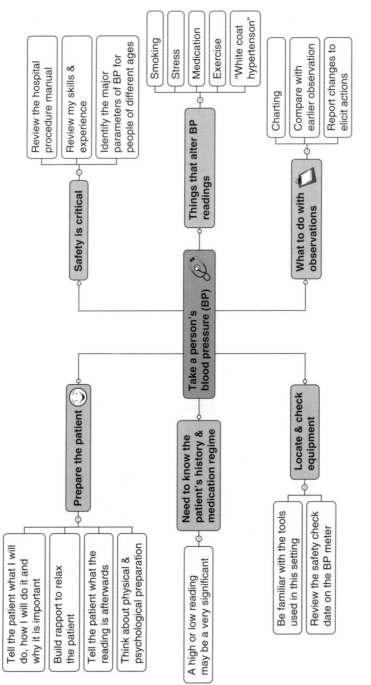

Figure 2.1 An example of the use of brainstorming for taking a blood pressure

have a go at using the technique in the explanation of the technique that follows next.

The technique

1. On a sheet of paper write a heading that indicates the broad area that you wish to explore, for example 'Nursing' or 'Counselling' or 'Community Care'.

2. Under that heading and in no particular order, jot down everything that comes to mind when you think about that word. Do not omit anything and do not censor any words, phrases or sentences. Everything is to be jotted down. Continue this process until you have either filled the page or you can think of nothing else to write. The process may take anything from five minutes to one hour. The process may also be carried out in a group setting; when one person is elected to act as 'scribe' and who writes down the associations that other group members call out.

3. Now look through the list of words and phrases and strike out any that are not immediately relevant. Be careful, though: you will be surprised how seemingly 'odd' ideas can lead you to a new perspective on the topic. This stage is a period of reflection on the 'free associations' that you have made earlier. It is the stage in which links start to be made between seemingly disparate ideas.

4. Finally, place your ideas and associations in an order of priority. In this way you bring structure to your thoughts. You may wish to develop a fairly elaborate system of headings and subheadings or you may prefer only to cluster together certain related ideas. Either way, you will end the exercise with a wide range of ideas from which to work. Sometimes, you will end up with a huge number of ideas; at other times you will reach one single conclusion and that conclusion will very often be your real priority – even, if you are lucky, your research question itself.

5. Return to this list of ideas and phrases regularly and keep all the paperwork involved. In this way you can have a second period of reflection on the material and trace the development of your ideas as they evolve.

6. If the brainstorming procedure does help in the generation of a research question or problem, you will need to spend further time in refining the question or problem. This will usefully be done in the company of another person who has had research experience.

SUGGESTED FURTHER READING IF YOU WANT TO LEARN MORE ABOUT BRAINSTORMING

de Bono, E. (1990) *Lateral Thinking: A Textbook of Creativity*. Harmondsworth: Penguin.

http://www.mindtools.com/brainstm.html

=========== **EXERCISE 2.1 CONTINUED** ===========

Now, using the brainstorming technique, take a large sheet of paper and brainstorm all the sorts of issues that you are interested in as possible fields or aspects of research. A typical list may (or may not) look like this:

- pressure sores
- stress in nurses
- stress in myself
- skill mixes
- interpersonal skills
- counselling skills
- care of the dying
- clinical governance
- hospital-acquired infections
- managing change

- practice development
- learning climate
- reflective practice
- arts in nursing
- clinical supervision
- overseas-trained nurses
- multicultural health assessment
- poverty and health
- nursing models: do they work?
- what are nursing models?

Notice, as the list above has developed, questions have begun to form. This is the beginning of the process of clarification of a possible research problem or question. Note that the last two items in the above list begin to narrow in focus. You will find it helpful to be as specific as you can when you come to framing your research question. We suggest that you work with your brainstorming and prioritization until you can frame your research problem or question in one sentence. Be warned – this is easier said than done.

Some negative and positive examples of research questions are offered below: some of them will lead to systematic and logical enquiry (the positive ones), the others will need further clarification. Look through the list and mark which ones you see as being positive and which as negative. When you have completed this task, go back to your own work and further refine the question or problem until you are sure that the statement is unambiguous, clear and addresses only a single issue. The list of positive and negative research question is as follows:

- How do nurses care for dying patients?

- Are nurses good at interpersonal skills?

- What interpersonal skills do nursing clinical leaders identify as being important in dealing with distressed relatives?

- How many patients on ward 'X' have sacral pressure sores of more than 2 cm in diameter?

- What factors in nursing are perceived by ward staff as stressful?

- What is the ratio of registered nursing staff to unlicensed care workers in this hospital?

- Evaluate the impact of using the Braden Scale to minimize pressure areas for bedridden patients.

What relevance do you think these problems have to your everyday work as a nurse? It is interesting to consider the degree to which research questions and problems arise out of everyday nursing practice and the degree to which they are 'generated' by the person who sets out to undertake a research project. Should all nursing research address practical issues or should some research be carried out to clarify theoretical issues?

Evaluation: Check your results through with a supervisor and discuss the difficulties of clarifying your own research question or problem. What are the constituents of a good research question? Were the research questions or problems clearly stated in the research projects you have read so far? Go back to one of them and try to extract such a question, issue or problem.

Ethical considerations

'Ethics' is concerned with issues of 'right and wrong' and 'good and bad'. The professional standards or codes for ethical conduct that guide nurses in clinical practice apply to nurses in the research context. As well, many government research funding bodies have guidelines that describe the requirements for ethical research.

SUGGESTED WEBSITES TO REVIEW DIFFERENT CODES AND STANDARDS FOR ETHICAL RESEARCH

http://www.anmc.org.au/userfiles/file/New%20Code%20of%20Ethics%20 for%20Nurses%20August%202008.pdf

http://www.rcn.org.uk/__data/assets/pdf_file/0013/236020/003138.pdf

http://www.nhmrc.gov.au/health_ethics/index.htm

http://www.mrc.ac.uk/Ourresearch/Ethicsresearchguidance/index.htm

http://www.esrc.ac.uk/ESRCInfoCentre/Images/ESRC_Re_Ethics_Frame_ tcm6-11291.pdf

http://www.wma.net/en/30publications/10policies/b3/index.html

In research, ethical questions must be asked at all stages of the process. It is important to continue to ask questions such as:

- Is it right that I am asking people these questions in the process of doing my research?

- Is what I am doing likely to harm anyone, physically, emotionally or socially?

- Are my questions worth asking? Are they appropriate and/or important?

- How do the potential benefits of the project outweigh the potential risks?

- Have I considered the impact my project might have from a range of perspectives?

We cannot assume that we have a right to undertake research or to ask questions of people, without gaining their permission or informed consent. To protect people's rights in this area, area health authorities and universities have ethics committees which ask that researchers submit a copy of their research proposal for assessment regarding its ethical status. You must be clear about the ethical requirements and procedures for the ethics committee that you will be submitting your proposal to for approval *before* you proceed beyond the planning stage with your research. Many ethics committees will have a standard form that has to be filled in and submitted with the research proposal. The ethics committee may also ask to interview you about your proposal.

It is important not to overlook ethical issues when planning research. It is essential to discuss any proposals that you have (particularly if they involve asking for patient's cooperation) with your supervisor(s). Many applications submitted to ethics committees are returned to the applicant requiring further work and refinements to satisfy the committee that the project meets appropriate ethical standards for research practice. Such delays can set you back weeks or even months so it is well worth the time to prepare a high quality application.

It is a good idea to have an informal chat with a member of the committee to explore in a relaxed way what you plan to do. This can help you to identify especially tricky areas like working with vulnerable groups, ensuring informed consent, privacy and respect for people. Many ethics committees categorize projects as low or high risk and respond accordingly. Do not assume that because you are a 'novice' researcher your project is low risk. Importantly a committee member can offer constructive advice on how to ensure that you deal with these areas in an ethically appropriate manner. You may be surprised how willing and open committee members are to share their expertise and it will save you time and energy if you get it right the first time.

Although ethics committee processes are important in providing some oversight to ensure ethical issues are addressed for a research project, at the end of the day the issue of ethical research relies on the integrity and professional behaviour of the researcher. The actions described in the research proposal and the ethics application that the researcher has stated will be done must be followed rigorously to ensure participants are protected, and that there is no misrepresentation of the research findings through fabrication, falsification or plagiarism at any stage of the research process.

SUGGESTED FURTHER READING ABOUT ETHICAL ISSUES IN RESEARCH

Polit, D. & Beck, C. (2010) *Essentials of Nursing Research: Appraising Evidence for Nursing Practice*. Philadelphia: Lippincott Williams & Wilkins, pp. 118–41.

Gerrish, K. & Lacey, A. (eds) (2009) *The Research Process in Nursing* (5th edn). Oxford: Blackwell Publishing, pp. 31–42.

Writing a research proposal

By the end of this section you will have discovered:

■ How to write a research proposal.

A research proposal is a detailed statement of what you intend to do, why you intend to do it and how you intend to go about it. It indicates both to you and anyone involved with your research both your ability to carry through the project and whether the design and methods you have selected are appropriate to the problem you have selected. The process of drawing up a research proposal can help you to further clarify your thoughts and methods. It is also necessary to give other people, outside of the project, the chance to examine your project and its methods. This is particularly true of those projects that required clearance through ethics committees. Any work involving patients will usually have to be considered by one or more such committees and those committees will always require you to submit a proposal. So too will anybody that is considering giving you an award or offering you research money.

The process of drawing up a research proposal is often one that takes considerable time to get right. You *will* have to rough out various drafts and the people that you submit the proposal to may ask you to make several changes. Do not be put off by this but continue to work through the proposal making the required changes. Do not refuse to make changes recommended to you by those to whom you submit your work. If you do, you run the risk of supervision or support being withdrawn rather rapidly. The drafting-feedback-redrafting approach usually leads to the development of a much tighter proposal.

In the next section you will find a structured outline for producing a research proposal. Note that this is only *one* way of drawing up such a proposal. Your school, college, university, awarding body or local health authority may have another format. Even if it does, the basic structure of the proposal will always be similar to this.

Guidelines for a research proposal

1. Title of the project
2. Name and designation of the researcher
3. Supervisor
4. Department (school or college)
5. Summary of the project (written for a lay person)

6. Statement of the problem

7. Aims and objectives of the project

8. Rationale for doing the research

9. Course of study being undertaken (if applicable)

10. Review of the pertinent literature

11. Research methods

12. Methods of analysis of data

13. Preparation of report

14. Ethical considerations

15. Costs involved (including itemized list and details of any funding bodies or details of self-funding)

16. Other considerations not covered in 1–12

17. Curriculum vitae of researcher (see the section 'Writing a curriculum vitae')

18. References.

SUGGESTED FURTHER READING

Gerrish, K. & Lacey, A. (eds) (2006) *The Research Process in Nursing* (5th edn). Oxford: Blackwell, pp. 123–37.

Kitson, A. (2002) Recognising relationships: Reflections on evidence-based practice. *Nursing Inquiry* 9(3): 179–86.

Punch, K. (2005) *Introduction to Social Research: Quantitative and Qualitative Approaches* (2nd edn). London: Sage Publishing, pp, 262–68.

EXERCISE 2.2

Aim of the exercise: To draw up a research proposal.

What to do: Make a word processing file with the research proposal outline above, and make notes about your own research under those headings. Then continue to refine the proposal until you are content that it is clear, detailed and complete. You may find it helpful to use the brainstorming technique again under each of the subheadings and then write the ideas out in sentences and paragraphs when you have finished.

Evaluation: Show your proposal to a supervisor and take note of any modifications that are suggested. After you have written the proposal, ask yourself the following questions:

- Is the proposal realistic? Have I the necessary skills to undertake this piece of research? Have I the time to carry it through? Do I know how to undertake the various stages?

- Is the proposal clear? Have I used simple, unambiguous language and avoided unnecessary jargon?

- Does the proposal require ethical approval and what particular ethical considerations need to be addressed?

- Can the proposal be converted into a realistic timeline with appropriate goals and sub-goals which take account of your other study/work commitments?

- Will the proposal be understandable by a reader who does not possess the technical language of nursing and other health professionals?

Always explain technical terms, especially if the proposal is going to be read by lay people or those unfamiliar with research. It can be helpful to ask someone who knows nothing about the topic to read your proposal and tell you if they understood what you have written. Remember that your proposal will be provisional and require further amendments as you develop your thoughts and ideas. Bear in mind, too, that you may have to modify your proposal further as you learn more about research and specific requirements of your chosen project. As we noted earlier, research can be a messy business and does not always go to plan. Sometimes, unexpected contingencies will force you to modify your plans. It is impossible to foreshadow everything that might happen in a research study involving humans but it is possible to anticipate some of the more obvious pitfalls by revisiting the questions below from time to time.

- Have I covered each aspect of the proposal thoroughly?

- Does the proposal paint a complete word picture of what I intend to do, how I intend to do it and why it is important?

- Can I anticipate any sections of the proposal which may cause others such as colleagues, patients, managers, or members of the ethics committee, to be concerned or to ask questions?

Always be prepared for questions from other people, especially from supervisors and ethics committees. If you do not know the answers to their questions do not worry – but make sure you find out later and then respond in person or send an email. Finding things out is the mark of a good researcher.

Writing a curriculum vitae

There are many occasions, including when you are preparing a research proposal, when you will be required to present a curriculum vitae (CV). This should be typed, and should set out your 'work/ study/ community life history' to date. Your CV gives the reader the opportunity to assess your suitability for undertaking the research you have planned. It also offers an insight into how you have studied and trained and the work that you have done to date. It is worthwhile investing time in the preparation of a CV and it is advisable to keep copies of it which can be updated from time to time. It is usual to divide the CV up into sections for clarity of presentation and ease of reading. Always keep a copy of your CV saved (and backed-up) on your computer and add to it as your circumstances change.

For examples of different styles search the internet using search headings such as 'examples of CVs'. You will find that there are many different formats that can be used depending on the circumstance and the requirements of the organization where you are submitting your CV.

Identifying constraints

By the end of this section you will have discovered:

■ What constraints are likely to affect your research?

================ **EXERCISE 2.3** ================

Aim of the exercise: To explore constraints as they apply to your project.

What to do: Sit on your own and write down on a sheet of paper (or better still create a word processing file) the headings contained Table 2.1. The structure of the table will allow you to identify any potential snags in your project and anything that may stand in the way of completing it. In the second column of the table, you are encouraged to use a problem-solving approach to identifying ways of dealing with the constraints that you have identified. You are then asked to plan action to help overcome any constraints. The process of doing the exercise will make the next stages of your project easier or indicate where some changes to the original plan may need to be made.

Table 2.1   Exploring possible constraints in your research project

Possible constraints	Suggestions to manage these	Actions
Brainstorm all possible constraints here. They may include such things as: ▪ Other people's attitudes ▪ Time factors ▪ Financial limitations ▪ Lack of specialist knowledge and skills about research.	Identify ideas for managing each constraint. Some constraints may be insurmountable but at least you will be prepared and you will be better able to plan what to do next.	Write in here realistic things to be done and how you will do them. It is also a good idea to check if the action has been successful or not. Don't assume that because you made a request to a line manager that others will be informed!

Evaluation: What constraints did you identify? If you identified too many or the constraints were too large you may have to rethink part of your project and reduce your expectations. Many people start out with enough ideas for three PhDs but only have six months to complete a small project well. Discuss your findings with your colleagues and with a supervisor and ask them to think about what they believe may be constraints in your project. Be prepared to accept criticism and be prepared to adapt your strategy. Do not become defensive. Good proposals require hard work and time. Actively seek out feedback from others. This is another exercise that you can return to at various stages throughout the research process in order to plan ahead.

At this stage, you may want to consider the question of pilot testing your plan. A pilot study (as we will discuss later in chapter 7) is a small study to enable you to discover whether your proposed plan works well in practice. Discuss with your supervisor whether this would be a good time to institute a pilot study. The pilot study can be an ideal way of uncovering practical and organizational problems. Once uncovered, these issues can be accounted for and your plan modified accordingly. However, a pilot study too will still require ethical approval if it involves other people or important information about people.

CONCLUSION

By now you should have prepared your initial proposal and be reasonably confident that you can develop this further after receiving feedback and carry it through. The more time that you spend in this process, the better. It is preferable to iron out as many problems as you can early on rather than to have to make substantial changes later on.

CHAPTER

Searching the Literature

AIMS OF THIS CHAPTER

- To explore literature resources;

- To discuss how to conduct a literature search;

- To consider how to review the literature critically;

- To encourage the writing of a literature review.

Introduction

This chapter focuses on the skills you will need in order to search for and then critically appraise literature relevant to your project. A systematic search of the work already carried out in your field of interest is necessary so that you are clear about what has and has not been done previously which identifies those areas that require further research. You need to be conscientious and organized. It is very easy to miss major areas of research on your topic or conversely to be swamped by the amount of information you uncover.

When you have completed the literature review, you will be able to:

- Identify the many sources where you may find research literature relevant to your topic.

- Critically review and summarize the previous research in your field of study.

- Identify important omissions in the work that has already been completed and design your study so that you are adding to the established body of knowledge – even in a small way.

- Have a better idea about what approaches and methods other researchers have used to study the area and be able to make an informed choice about the appropriateness of different procedures.

Finally, it is worth noting that you must continue to search the literature throughout all the stages of the research process. Your field of study is constantly changing. You must keep up to date.

Exploring the literature resources

By the end of this section you will have discovered:

- Where to find information about previous work related to your field of study;

- The accessibility of using these sources from the points of view of time, energy and cost.

There are many sources of literature available to you. These include libraries for books and journals, electronic searching using library databases, e-journals, search engines on the web, and using reference lists from articles on your topic which will lead you to other research reports in your area of interest. As well there is another source which is termed grey literature which comprises information about your topic, which may not be referenced in any of the sources above but can provide you with significant information. These can include conference papers, unpublished government or health service reports and pamphlets. This grey literature requires some detective work to find and can involve searching on the internet, contacting interest groups or government departments.

EXERCISE 3.1

Aim of the exercise: To identify literature resources.

What to do: Draw three concentric circles on a page (see the example in Figure 3.1). The inner circle represents literature resources that are immediately available (e.g. your own books, journals, etc.). The middle circle represents those resources that are available within reasonably easy reach (e.g. school of nursing library, hospital library, public library, friends, colleagues, etc.). The outer circle represents those resources that

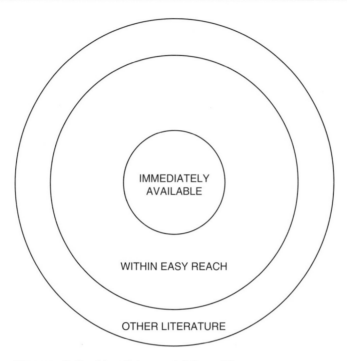

IMMEDIATELY
AVAILABLE

WITHIN EASY REACH

OTHER LITERATURE

Figure 3.1   Identifying availability of literature resources

are available through rather more application (e.g. the internet – library bibliographic databases, e-journals, search engines such as Google, Yahoo or Google scholar and inter-library loan scheme, etc.). Personalize this diagram so that it becomes a source of reference for you when you do your literature searching. Add to it as you discover new sources of information. Keep it with you throughout your research project. You will often need it. Also, keep a list of the libraries and resource centres that you have visited and the sections in those departments that you have explored. In this way, you become more systematic in your search and avoid unnecessary repetition.

Evaluation: Go through the information contained in the three circles and identify which sources you are using at present. Write down on a sheet of paper those sources that you need more information about and write down those sources that you will use in the coming weeks. Do any of the sources charge for their services? If so, have you budgeted for this? Are any of the sources likely to take considerable time to respond to your request? If so, can you account for this in planning your work? If not, would it be better to seek this information from another source? Finally, do you really need this information: is it vital to your project? If you have doubts about this, talk to your supervisor about this piece of information.

Much time can be lost searching out esoteric and obscure papers that only distantly relate to the project. Keep it simple: start with the obvious.

Finding relevant literature

By the end of this section you will have discovered:

- How to find literature and information as part of your research project;
- How to keep records of the literature you find.

Having identified the different sources of literature the next step in the process is to learn techniques to find the literature. This process can be time consuming and frustrating as you search for clues, narrow your search and sift for what is relevant and not relevant. The first thing you must do is identify what you are actually looking for. What is your topic area, what particularly in your topic area are you seeking more information about and what limits do you want to put in place in terms of the search? This process is called developing your research strategy.

SUGGESTED READING: BOTH THESE AUTHORS DESCRIBE SUCCINCTLY HOW TO DEVELOP A RESEARCH STRATEGY

Beecroft, C., Rees, A., & Booth, A. (2009) Finding the evidence. In K. Gerrish & A. Lacey (eds) *The Research Process in Nursing*. Oxford: Blackwell Publishing, pp. 95–7.

Polit, D. & Beck, C. (2010). *Essentials of Nursing Research: Appraising Evidence for Nursing Practice*. Philadelphia: Lippincott Williams & Wilkins, pp. 173–81.

Remember not to be too narrow in your search for relevant literature. A good starting point is the library. Most will have 'beginner guides' to get you started on how and where to search for resources and if things get tricky ask one of the helpful librarians dedicated to the 'health' area. Many libraries will run courses to help you find the most efficient and effective ways of finding materials. Consider using materials from the social, biological and behavioural sciences, as well as those in nursing and midwifery. When you begin to search the large array of research databases available you will be struck by the speed and range of articles that may present themselves. On some occasions you may generate hundreds of papers yet none of them might seem wholly relevant. This highlights the need to identify very specific search terms and to link these together so that fewer and more relevant papers can be distilled from a general search of the databases.

EXERCISE 3.2

Aim of the exercise: To find specific information from different types of resources available.

Planning stage: For the purposes of this exercise you will be looking for information about your topic of interest. Allow yourself plenty of time to complete the exercise and make notes of what you do, as you go.

There are four parts to this exercise.

Part one: Manual search for books

Go to a library which contains a selection of books and journals on nursing. Ask the librarian to explain the cataloguing system to you. Find the bookshelves that may have books dealing with your topic and scan the book titles for anything you think may be relevant. Look at the contents pages of these books and see if you can find relevant information. Review quickly and see if there are relevant sections you may like to make notes or photocopy the section. Review the references in the book to give you clues for more information. If there is relevant information you may like to photocopy this section as well. You do need to note that if you are photocopying from journals and books that there are copyright rules that will apply. Check with the librarian to ensure that you are complying with these. Make sure you note down all the details of the book for the future (the author, title, date and place of publication, edition and class number which tells where the book can be found in the library – this helps you to avoid looking up the details again).

Part two: Manual search for Journals

Using the library catalogue find journals that the library has copies of that may have information about your topic. Review the contents page for relevant articles. Scan any relevant articles and if there are relevant sections you may like to make notes or photocopy the article. Review the references at the end of the article to give you clues for more information. If there is relevant information you may like to photocopy this section as well; just remember the copyright rules referred to above. Make sure you note down all the details of the journal, the article and the author for the future. If you make a photocopy of an article make a note that you have this and where it is filed.

Part three: Electronic search for bibliographic databases

Using a computer linked to the hospital or university library you now need to search the electronic bibliographic databases that the library has access to. Ask the librarian to give you some advice on how to access these databases. Most databases have the facility for you to search key-words, phrases, subjects or authors. There is also normally the facility to limit your search to specific types of search (e.g. full text, abstract, peer review, within certain time frames etc....). Another feature known as Boolean operators provides the opportunity when you are searching to use 'and, or, not' terms to combine or restrict searches. Using these functions enter your search terms in the database/s that you are using to search. You may need to do this many times so you can limit the search results to a manageable size. You will need to scan the result list for relevant articles, review these and 'save' those that will be relevant. You can also look at the list of the references at the end of the relevant articles which can give you another source of information.

By now you will probably have a fair bit of information. The most impor-tant point here is to ensure you have a method of keeping track of the information you find. If you have downloaded PDF (Portable Document File) copies of articles make a note of these and where they are filed. More about this is detailed further in this chapter.

Part four: Electronic search: search engines/relevant websites

This final part of the exercise requires you to use the internet to search for information using different search engines such as Google, Yahoo and Google Scholar. Choose one of these and write in some of your search terms. (Some search engines do allow you to use Boolean operators to limit or extend your search.) You will probably find that, because search engines trawl a large amount of data, unless you limit your search you will come up with a result list that is far too large for you to review. It takes time and practice but you should keep refining your search terms until you have a manageable result list. Again a helpful librarian is a good person to help you to refine your search. This type of search may well also help with your search for grey literature as often you will find useful links and websites that will not appear in the database search. An important point here is that you must be very discerning when selecting search engines and websites in terms of the veracity and the quality of the information you find.

Evaluation: What, if any, problems did you have with the different types of literature searching? Were you overwhelmed with the amount of informa-tion? If so, how did you reduce this to a manageable level? How did you keep track of all of the information you found?

SUGGESTED READING

The following readings give different descriptions of the processes that you have just undertaken. You may find that these different views help you understand the processes better.

Bell, J. (2005) *Doing Your Research Project: A Guide for First-Time Researchers in Education, Health and Social Science* (4th edn). Berkshire: Open University Press, pp. 79–89.

Polit, D. & Beck, C. (2010) *Essentials of Nursing Research: Appraising Evidence for Nursing Practice*. Philadelphia: Lippincott Williams & Wilkins, pp. 173–81.

iTunesU - http://www.apple.com/education/guidedtours/itunesu.html

Tools for preparing for a literature review at: http://www.gwu.edu/~litrev/

Keeping track of your references

By the end of this section you will have discovered:

■ How to keep a record of what you read;

■ How to organize these records.

Most of us at some time or another have been in the situation where we can remember some details of something we have read about a certain topic but we need to check further details. However, we cannot remember where we read it, who wrote it or what newspaper, journal, book or electronic resource it was in. Many hours/days /weeks are wasted while we search for the elusive reference. If we are lucky we finally find it, if not, it becomes an irritant that continues to annoy us for a long time. So, one of the most crucial things that you need to master as a researcher is to find a method of keeping track of what you read. It does not matter whether your intention is to limit your research to undertaking searches for evidence to support your clinical or management practice, or to have continuing involvement in formal research projects, over time you will read and access many resources. You must have a method of being able to retrieve your references in an effective manner.

Depending on your own personal style there are several methods which you can use. Some people prefer to keep manual files using index cards, notebooks or sheets of paper filed in some orderly manner. Manual methods have the advantage that as long as you have a pen and paper it is always accessible wherever you happen to be reading your resource. However, the disadvantage is that you need to be disciplined in developing a filing system so that as your list of resources grows you can actually find the information you require in the future.

Other people prefer to create electronic files of their resource information using Word or Excel files or specific bibliographic software like EndNote® or Refworks. Each method has it advantages and disadvantages. There are many advantages to this approach to storing references. First, you can add new ones to the file very easily. Second, you can easily 'cut and paste' references from your list straight into your essay or project. Third, the whole system is very easy to use and administer. If you feel that you will be collecting huge numbers of references, this system may suit you. The disadvantage is that your computer may not be accessible when you are reading and so information is not recorded immediately and then you never get round to entering on your electronic filing system.

It does not matter which system you use as long as you adopt and continue to use a process of keeping track of your resources.

SUGGESTED READING

The excerpt from the following book provides further insight into the need to keep track of your literature resources in a systematic way.

Bell, J. (2008) Doing Your Research Project: A Guide for First-Time Researchers in Education, Health and Social Science (4th edn). Berkshire: Open University Press, pp. 68–77.

EXERCISE 3.3

Aims of the exercise: To demonstrate how you can make useful notes from what you read, and how to organize these so you can keep track of what you have read.

There are two parts to this exercise.

Part one: Manual reference system

Equipment required: Index cards (13 x 7.5 cms) and a box for filing the cards in, or a notebook, or sheets of paper, and a pen.

Find the following article either manually by going to your library or electronically using bibliographic databases:

Zambas, S. (2010) Purpose of the systematic physical assessment in everyday practice: Critique of the 'Sacred Cow'. *Journal of Nursing Education* 49(6): 305–9.

Now attempt to answer the following questions:

(a)   What is the argument that Zambas puts forward for questioning the teaching systematic physical assessment to nursing students?

(b)   What is Zambas suggesting as an alternative?

(c)   What is the rationale that Zambas offers for the alternative?

Once you have read the article and answered the questions you will need to make an accurate record of what the authors have said in support of your answers. Details about the sources of your literature, and any direct quotes that you may find useful are required so that your project can be written up and referenced accurately. We recommend that you use the following system.

Prepare your notes on what you have just read using index cards, a notebook or a sheet of paper in the format illustrated in Figure 3.2. By all means tailor the layout to suit your own needs but once you have settled on a format, stick to it. Always carry some index cards, a notebook or sheets of paper around with you; so that when you find a new and relevant reference, you can make notes about it, there and then.

You will need to develop a filing system so that you will be able to ret-erive the notes easily. Whichever manual systen you adopt you will need to keep an index of each note as you make it and the date it was written so you will be able to find it in the future. We have also found it helpful to make a note of where you found the particular resource or where you are keeping the hard copy. This means that if required it is much quicker to go back to the original resource.

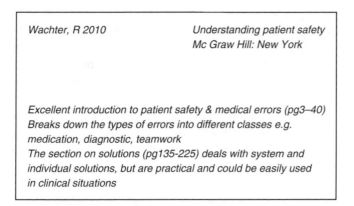

Figure 3.2   Keeping track of references using a manual
system

Part two: Computerised reference databases

A manual reference system will help you to keep your records up-to-date and accurate. Of course there are several computer programs available to help store, search and use your references efficiently. If you plan on doing a substantial project then use one of these. If your project is small, then the card system will suffice and can easily be converted into a simple word processing or spreadsheet file later.

Using the articles and information you reviewed above simply open a word processing file and then put your references into it, in the form of paragraphs, as you collect them. If your word processor has a 'sorting' facility, it does not matter what 'order' you type them in. Once you have put in new references, you get the program to sort the entire list into alphabetical order. Here is an example of what a file might look like:

File: Notes on Narrative:

Fraser, M., (2006) Outsider-witness practices in developing community with women who have experienced child sexual assault. *The International Journal of Narrative Therapy and Community Work* 3: 52–8.

Describes the West Street Centre's community forum days, and the narrative practices and foundations that went into the planning of these days

Sax, P. (2006) Developing preferred stories of identity as reflective practitioners. *Journal of Systemic Therapies* 25(4): 59–72.

The assignment 'Preferred Stories of Identity' was offered as a way in which to teach students the five aspects of narrative practice. Excerpts of students' work are shown throughout the paper.

The second approach is to use a ready written database program such as EndNote®, Reference Manager or Refworks. These bibliographical database programs are specially written for recording references and allow you to download details about the articles or books that you find in research literature or the library catalogue. These references can then be 'inserted' into word processed documents as research proposals, plans and reports without any need for re-typing. These programs do require some investment and commitment in time to learn to use them. However the advantages of being able to insert references directly into your word documents in whichever referencing style that might be required, and the search mechanism embedded in within them provides a level of efficiency that manual methods and simple word files lack.

Figure 3.3 shows a screen shot of EndNote® with information that we gathered in part one of the exercise.

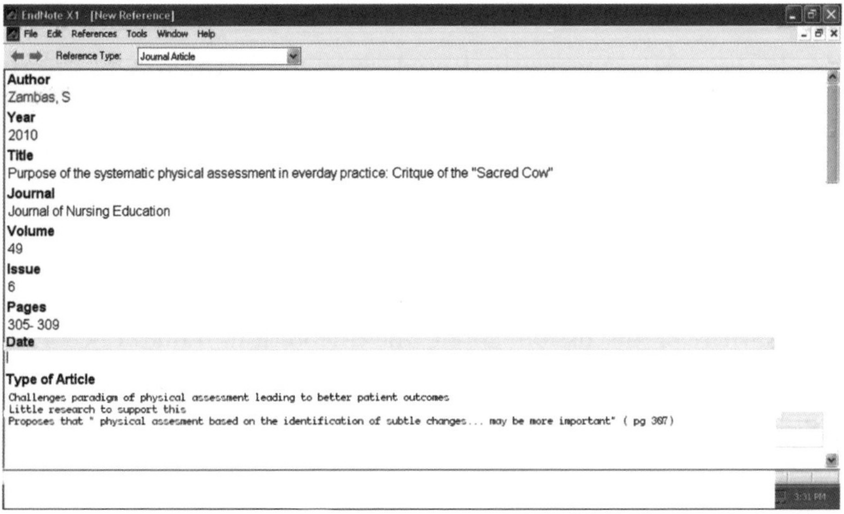

Figure 3.3   Keeping track of references electronically

Source: Endnote®, © Copyright 2011 Thomson Reuters. Reproduced with permission.

Critically reviewing the literature

By the end of this section you will have discovered:

■ How to review what you read critically.

Guidelines for evaluating research reports

As you start looking at the literature concerning your project you will probably find that there is an enormous amount of literature available. Deciding on the relevance and quality of what you are reading is an important skill to develop. The following guidelines will help you to ask evaluative questions about that research. The guidelines will also help you to firm up your ideas about problems, methods and analytical techniques in your own research project.

1. The Research Problem

   ■ Is the problem clearly stated?

   ■ Is the problem researchable?

   ■ Does the problem relate directly to nursing?

2. The Literature Review

   ■ Is the review of the literature relevant to the topic?

   ■ Is it comprehensive?

- How current are the sources of literature?

- Is the referencing method used correctly? Is the review laid out logically?

- Is a summary offered at the end of the review that spells out implications for the present study?

3. Design of the Study

- Is there a statement of the overall design of the study?

- Is there a discussion about the theoretical framework of the study?

- If hypotheses are offered, are they unambiguous and clearly stated?

- Is there a clear description of:

    (a) What the researcher planned to do?

    (b) What the researcher did?

    (c) How the researcher did it?

- Are relevant technical terms defined clearly?

4. Data Collection

- Is the data collection method described clearly?

- Does the researcher justify the use of her method?

- Is the sample discussed in terms of relevance and size?

- Are the instruments used for data collection clearly described?

- Are the issues of reliability and validity addressed? (These are discussed in chapter 6 of this book.)

- Is there a clear description of what the researcher did when she collected the data?

5. Data Analysis

- Are the methods of analysis appropriate for the data?

- Are those methods clearly described?

- Is the presentation of findings clearly laid out (in tables, graphs, pie charts, etc.)?

- Is there adequate discussion of the results and findings?

6. Conclusions and Recommendations

- Are the conclusions that the researcher makes justified?

- Are the conclusions linked sufficiently with the researcher's original purpose?

- Are the recommendations practical?

- Has the researcher discussed the implications for further research?

- Has the researcher discussed the limitations of the study?

SUGGESTED FURTHER READING

This will give you other perspectives about how to review critically the literature that you are reading:

http://library.ucsc.edu/ref/howto/literaturereview.html

http://www.deakin.edu.au/library/findout/research/litrev.php

Smith, K. (2008) Building upon existing evidence to shape future research endeavors. *American Journal of Health System Pharmacy* 65: 1767–74.

Reviewing other literature

Apart from reviewing research reports, you will want to read other sorts of literature including: theoretical discussion in journals and books, biographical literature, discussion of methodology and technique, textbooks, policy documents, official reports and sometimes fiction.

As you read, consider the following:

- Are arguments expressed clearly?

- Are they substantiated by either:

  (a) Reference to research or

  (b) Rational argument?

- Are the assumptions underlying an argument spelt out?

- Are the limitations of a particular argument identified?

- Does the author have a particular position to state which blinds him to other possibilities?

- Is the discussion balanced and informed or is it polemical?

- If rational argument is used, does it flow in a logical and ordered manner?

■ Are the arguments relevant to your subject area?

■ Does the author use technical terms and if so does he explain what he means by his use of them?

■ Could you summarize the main points of argument?

■ Have other authors that you have read expressed different views? Could you summarize them?

■ Do you agree with what the author says? If so, why? If not, why?

This is not an exhaustive list of possible issues to be explored when reading literature other than research reports but it will help you to evaluate what you read and to become more critical of your reading.

──────────────── **EXERCISE 3.4** ────────────────

Aim of the exercise: To explore styles of critical literature reviewing.

Read the literature review sections of the following two articles. Compare the two styles of reviewing and note how each author uses references to other work. Note, too, whether or not they are critical of other people's work. It is important that reviews of the literature do not become lists of other people's research or theories.
   Points to look for as you read:

■ Does the author break the review up into sections?

■ Does he/she question the methodology of previous research?

■ Does he/she challenge the assumptions that previous writers make?

■ Do you understand the points that are made?

■ Is the review interesting?

■ How recent is the literature referred to in the review?

■ Is the review balanced: 'critical' does not just mean 'criticize'.

■ Does the author have a particular axe to grind: philosophical, political, ideological?

Keep asking questions about what you are reading. Do not take what the writer says for granted. Challenge what is written and look for reasons for and explanations of the writer's arguments. To do this is to begin the process of critical evaluation. Note, however, that to be 'critical' is not only to pick holes in the work nor to see it only in a negative light. To be critical is also to be able to discriminate between the 'good' as well as the 'bad' parts of the work.

The two articles for consideration are:

http://eprints.qut.edu.au/263/1/SIMPSON_CRITICAL_THINKING.PDF

http://www.journalofadvancednursing.com/docs/0309–2402.2003.02853.x.pdf

Make notes on the content of the two papers and record these and the references using either the manual or electronic system you have adopted. In this way you will reinforce the habit of keeping notes and recording the references of your reading.

Evaluation: Read through your notes, consider your summaries and then ask a colleague to read one of the papers and discuss your individual views. Note how different people's perceptions of the same paper can vary considerably.

Writing a literature review

By the end of this section you will have discovered:

■ How to write your own literature review.

Writing a literature review

The point about writing up a literature review is not simply to list all the books and papers that you have read about the particular topic in question but to do so *critically*. You also need to *organize* the review under a range of headings. It is important that a literature review should 'flow' and that it takes the reader through a series of sections that are logical and orderly. The overall aim of the literature review is to place your piece of research in context. It should answer the following questions:

■ What research has been done prior to this study?

■ Why is this field of study of interest?

■ What are some of the problems associated with this field?

■ How is the field organized?

■ What are the main theories, arguments, research designs, modes of analysis used in the field?

■ How does all this link with the *larger* field of nursing?

■ What new issues, needing to be addressed, have emerged from your search of the literature?

■ What are the recommended approaches for dealing with these issues?

A good literature review should take into account the following points.

- It should be comprehensive and up-to-date.
- It should be clearly structured with good use made of headings and subheadings.
- It should be a *critical* account of previous work carried out in the field.
- It should be appropriately and accurately referenced.

SUGGESTED READING

Bernardo, L. M., Matthews, J. T. Kaufmann, J. A. & Yang, K. (2008) Promoting critical appraisal of the research literature: A workshop for school nurses. *The Journal of Continuing Education in Nursing* 39(10): 461–7.

Nkowane, A. M. & Saxena, S. (2004) Opportunities for an improved role for nurses in psychoactive use: Review of the literature. *International Journal of Nursing Practice* 10: 102–10.

Smith, K. (2008) Building upon existing evidence to shape future research endeavours. *American Society of Health-System Pharmacists* 65: 1767–74.

=============== **EXERCISE 3.5** ===============

Aim of the exercise: To undertake a short literature review.

Planning stage: Identify a topic of your choice. Identify the literature resources relevant to your chosen area. *What to do*: Go to your library and find ten articles or books related to your chosen subject area. Make a summary of each of these either using your manual or electronic recording system, which should, of course, contain full details of the references. Then write a critical review of the ten articles of not more than 500–1000 words.

Evaluation: Choose one of the following options:

(a) Show the review to your lecturer or supervisor;

(b) Ask friends or colleagues to read and comment on it;

(c) Share the review with a group of colleagues who have also undertaken the exercise.

You have now carried out one stage of the research process.

CONCLUSION

You should now be able to collect information relating to your area of interest and record the reference details as well as the key findings and issues that you found as you studied the information. You should also be developing an awareness of how to read and write a 'critical' literature review. Continue to read around these subjects and then move on to the next chapter in which we explore different approaches to research methodology. The skills learnt in this stage of the research process will be called upon time and time again throughout the development of your project.

Approaches to Research Methodology

4

- To list the distinguishing characteristics between quantitative and qualitative approaches to research;

- To discriminate between descriptive and experimental research;

- To identify the problems associated with subjectivity and objectivity;

- To help you consider the influence of your beliefs and philosophy in your choice of approach or series of approaches.

Introduction

As we have noted, there are different approaches to thinking about and doing research. Sometimes it is useful to count and categorize things. At other times it is instructive to find out how people perceive things. This chapter explores some differences between various approaches to research. The temptation to polarize thinking into approaches being 'either/or', is a strong one. We hope that in looking at the different concepts involved in this chapter you will come to see the various approaches as complimentary rather than competitive.

Before we begin we should acknowledge that the use of some terms or research jargon is essential to help communicate ideas quickly and efficiently. At the same time, technical terms and phrases such as methodology, methods, approach, strategy and design can cause confusion as different writers use them in different ways. In this book research methodology refers to the broad approaches referred to as quantitative (things you can count and do statistics on), qualitative (texts or words that can be interpreted) or a combination of the two. Research design refers to the overall description of a particular study from the beginning to the end, and method describes the processes of how you will collect data.

SUGGESTED READING

These authors describe the different characteristics of qualitative and quantitative research. These readings will also help you with the activities throughout this chapter.

Borbasi, S., Jackson, D. & Langford, R. (2008) *Navigating the Maze of Nursing Research* (2nd edn). Marrackville: Elsevier, pp. 103–78.

Creswell, J. W. (2009) *Research Design: Qualitative, Quantitative, and Mixed Methods Approaches* (3rd edn). London: Sage, pp. 145–202.

Coolican, H. (2009) *Research Methods and Statistics in Psychology* (5th edn). London: Hodder Arnold, pp. 1–27 and 222–46.

Gerrish, K. & Lacey, A. (eds) (2006) *The Research Process in Nursing* (5th edn). Oxford: Blackwell, pp. 163–71.

The differences between quantitative and qualitative research

By the end of this section you will have discovered:

- What the two words mean;

- How various writers define the distinction between the two in research;

- Some examples of quantitative and qualitative research.

EXERCISE 4.1

Aim of the exercise: To define the words 'quantitative' and 'qualitative' and to identify the differences between the two approaches to methodology.

There are three parts to this exercise.

Part one

Read three of the references referred to above. Find out how those writers use the words quantitative and qualitative. Then look up those words in a dictionary and notice any difference in usage between the dictionary and the usage of words in the research literature. How useful are dictionary definitions when considering the ways words are used in research? Discuss the various definitions of the two approaches and consider how you may draw out characteristics that distinguish the two approaches from one another.

Part two

Now that you have defined the two approaches, look through and read sections of books on research and nursing research in the list above and complete the grid outlined in Figure 4.1. The grid offers you certain criteria for distinguishing between the practical differences between the two approaches. It also asks you to find three examples of quantitative and three examples of qualitative research from the nursing research literature. If you are working in a group, in your plenary session, try to think of other ways in which the two methods differ.

Characteristics	**Quantitative research**	**Qualitative research**
Purpose of the study		
Sample size		
Data collection methods		
Data analysis methods		
Method of presenting findings		
Three examples from the nursing literature		

Figure 4.1   Grid for comparing approaches

Part three

Now discuss these lists with a colleague or with the group that you are working with and compare what they have to say about the differences between the two approaches and your own work. Is it possible to make a clear distinction between the two? What types of research problems lend themselves to the different approaches? Have you managed to locate any nursing research studies that have used both approaches? If so, what particular aspects of these stand out?

Quantitative research

Although definitions of quantitative research vary, quantitative approaches usually incorporate some or all of the following features:

- Adopts an underlying philosophy of *positivism*. This is a word you should look up and be clear about.

- Attempts to establish or test *laws* and general principles.

- Counts things and uses statistics to make sense of the data that are gathered.

- Makes use of experiments and develops hypotheses to test relationships or causality between the issues/items being studied or to give an objective description, prediction or explanation of some aspect of study.

- Uses objective laboratory tests, psychometric scales or structured tests, processes, and instruments to gather and measure the data.

- Uses deductive reasoning (working from the general to the particular) to make sense of the analysis of the data.

- Employs validity and reliability tests to demonstrate objectivity.

Qualitative research

Although definitions of qualitative research vary, qualitative approaches usually incorporate some or all of the following features:

- Adopts a phenomenological perspective. This is another term that you should look up and become familiar with.

- Attempts to investigate personal subjective understanding and personal meaning attached to peoples' experiences.

- Uses small samples.

- Is concerned with *interpretation* rather than *quantification*.

- Uses inductive reasoning (working the particular case to the general) to interpret the findings of the data analysis.

- Often involves in-depth interviews, observation and the exploration of personal documents to study the experiences and understandings of people in a specific context.

- Uses different tests for reliability and validity to demonstrate the accuracy and authenticity of the process.

Mixed method research

What you may have found when you have been reading research reports is that some research uses a combination of quantitative and qualitative approaches. This use of some aspects of both types of approach is called mixed method research. There are advantages to combining both approaches when the research requires data that provide different perspectives on a problem or issue under investigation. This can limit the weaknesses of a single approach when trying to understand a complex problem and in health research many of the issues we explore may be quite complex with no single or straightforward solution.

If, for example, we were investigating the prevalence of pressure ulcers on a specific ward then a quantitative approach would probably be the appropriate approach. If we want to understand the impact on patients' lives and return to wellbeing when they develop pressure ulcers then a qualitative approach would probably be the choice. But, if we were comparing the prevalence of pressure ulcers in diabetic surgical patients with orthopaedic surgical patients and also investigating if the impact on patients' lives is different for these two groups, then a mixed method would probably be the most appropriate.

SUGGESTED READING FOR AN OVERVIEW OF MIXED METHODS RESEARCH

Creswell, J. & Plano-Clark, V. (2011) *Designing and Conducting Mixed Methods Research*. California: Sage, pp. 1–18.

Descriptive and experimental research

By the end of this section you will have discovered:

- The differences between descriptive and experimental research.

============================== **EXERCISE 4.2** ==============================

Aim of the exercise: To identify the differences between descriptive and experimental research.

What to do: Read the following four research reports which illustrate some different approaches to doing research:

Burnard, P. & Morrison, P. (2005) Nurses' perceptions of their interpersonal skills: A descriptive study using six category intervention analysis. *Nurse Education Today* 25: 612–17.

Edvardsson, D. (2009) Balancing between being a person and being a patient – a qualitative study of wearing patient clothing. *International Journal of Nursing Studies* 46: 4–11.

Day, J., Higgins, I. & Koch, T. (2009) The process of practice redesign in delirium care for hospitalised older people: A participatory action research study. *International Journal of Nursing Studies* 46: 13–22.

Levett-Jones, T., Lathlean, J., Higgins, I. & McMillan, M. (2008/9) The duration of clinical placements: A key influence on nursing students' experience of belongingness. *Australian Journal of Advanced Nursing* 26(2): 8–16.

Now answer the following questions:

■ What methods did each of the studies use?

■ What sort of information was collected in each of the studies? How was the data analysed?

■ What, if any, generalizations were made by the researchers?

Now read the next section, 'Descriptive and experimental research', which identifies some differences in approach between descriptive and experimental research. Which type of approach was used in the four studies?

Descriptive and experimental research

There are many differences between descriptive and experimental research and they often depend on differences of belief about the nature of people. For example, a person drawn to experimental research may believe that there are numerous similarities between people or that people's behaviour is causally determined. On the other hand, a person drawn to descriptive research may be more interested in just describing a place, situation or environment, believing that what is important in research is to note people's varying perceptions of the world and how they choose to interact with it. What we believe about the world will affect how we study it. Our beliefs about the nature of the world and of the people that inhabit it will affect:

■ The sorts of questions we ask;

■ The way we approach planning our research;

■ The sorts of research methods we use;

■ The way we interpret the data we collect;

■ The conclusions we draw from our findings.

Points of debate in research

For a number of years, there has been a debate about the pros and cons of quantitative and qualitative approaches to research. Some have seen this as a debate about *method* – about how to *do* research. Others have argued that it is a debate about what assumptions we make about human beings. The debate, however, is broader than just the quantitative/qualitative divide (and sometimes this is *not* a divide at all: as discussed above some writers and researchers have argued that it is possible and desirable to *combine* the approaches into a mixed methods approach). Hammersley (1992) offers a useful list of some of the points that are often raised when people argue about different approaches to research. The list may be useful in debates that *you* have about the topic:

1. Qualitative versus quantitative data;

2. The investigation of natural versus artificial settings;

3. A focus on meanings rather than on behaviour;

4. Adoption or rejection of natural science as a model;

5. An inductive versus a deductive approach;

6. Identifying cultural patterns as against seeking scientific laws;

7. Idealism versus realism.

When you reviewed this list did you find that there were terms that were unfamiliar? If so check back in this chapter and review the suggested readings. It would also be useful to see how many of the terms you can match up with your responses to the Grid for comparing approaches that you completed in Exercise 4.1. It is also a good idea to keep a record of any new technical terms you come across in your reading – it will save you having to look these up again on future occasions.

Subjectivity and objectivity in research

By the end of this section you will have discovered:

■ Some of the differences between subjectivity and objectivity;

■ Some of the problems associated with these two concepts.

━━━━━━━━━━━━━━━ **EXERCISE 4.3** ━━━━━━━━━━━━━━━

Aim of the exercise: To explore the problems of subjectivity and objectivity.

What to do:

1. Look up the words 'subjectivity' and 'objectivity' in a good dictionary (what do you class as 'good' in this context?) Then look at some books on research and read about how researchers have battled with the notions of subjectivity and objectivity.

2. With your colleagues, sit and write individual descriptions of the room you are in at present. Aim at writing about one page.

3. Read out your reports and decide:

   ■ whose description was most accurate?

   ■ whose was most objective?

   ■ whose was most interesting?

   ■ whose was most different to all the others?

   ■ whose was most appealing to the group and why?

   ■ whose was the least appealing and why?

   Now hold a discussion on the topic of subjectivity and objectivity and try to answer the following questions:

■ How can you be objective in research?

■ Do you need to be?

■ If so, why?

■ Is objectivity possible when you observe peoples' behaviour?

■ Is there a place in research for the subjective report?

■ If so, what is that place?

■ Are there particular aspects of nursing which lend themselves to more quantitative or more qualitative studies?

Read through a research report and note the degree to which the researcher has addressed the issue of objectivity. A useful paper, here, is:

Golafshani, N. (2003) Understanding reliability and validity in qualitative research. *The Qualitative Report* 8(4): 597–607.

The researcher's choice of methodology

As you have worked through this chapter you will have begun to address some of the complexities and ambiguities of the process of doing research. Although the type of research question will ultimately determine whether a quantitative, qualitative or mixed approach is most suitable, even before you decide on a research question, the way you think and act, and your own personal philosophy will affect your choice of research area and what sort of research questions you want to tackle. So, when making decisions about which research approach to use, you need to appreciate how your own beliefs about human beings and how you view the world influence this decision. You cannot detach yourself from your area of study to the degree that you look on as an objective and detached observer.

The following exercise helps you to think about these two issues.

By the end of this section you will have discovered:

- More about yourself.

- More about how your own beliefs about people and the world influence the way that you do research.

=============== **EXERCISE 4.4** ===============

Aim of the exercise: To explore individual beliefs about the person and about research.

The activity can be carried out alone or with a group of other people. Allow yourself plenty of time to complete the exercise and make notes of what you do, as you go. If you work with friends or colleagues, decide whether you will all carry out similar tasks or you will divide up the work between you.

What to do:

(a) Take a few sheets of paper and write out, in note form, your beliefs about how people are. For instance, you may or may not believe some of the following and may wish to make notes about how you agree or disagree with the statements. Write the piece fairly quickly; do not worry about 'style' and do not feel that the piece has to be an academic paper.

Some of the statements you may wish to agree or disagree with are:

- People are a product of their childhoods.

- A person's personality is shaped by society.

- A person is born with a certain personality.

- People are totally responsible for the way they are.

- God is responsible for the way people are.

- People can change themselves in fundamental ways.

- Most people are similar to most other people.

- We can measure people's behaviour.

- What a person does tells us what sort of person he is.

- People are basically aggressive by nature.

- People are born 'good': society corrupts them.

- People are born 'bad': they have to learn to be good.

- Events are causally linked.

- There is no absolute way of determining causality.

- All theories about people are open to question.

- People are subject to certain laws of human nature.

- People can make choices about all aspects of their lives.

(b) If you are working in a group, discuss your writing and your beliefs about the nature of the person with your colleagues. Then go through the paper and turn each of your statements into a question. Thus, if you have written: People are free to choose their lives, raise the question 'Are people free to choose their lives?' In this way, you begin to think critically about your own core beliefs and assumptions about people. Try, if you can, to argue against each of the questions and thus identify arguments that oppose your views.

(c) Now write out a short report of what you think are the functions and uses of research. Some of the things you may want to consider include the following:

- To add to the body of knowledge;

- To develop a greater understanding of people and the world;

- To attempt to predict the future;

- To enhance the environment;

- To contribute to other people's wellbeing;

- To create more interest in research, in the researcher;

- To disprove some theory;

- To test a theory;

- To understand another person's point of view;

- To inform practice;

- To satisfy course requirements;

- To challenge other people's theories or views of the world;

- To get a better job;

- To stretch yourself academically;

- To enhance your status.

If you are working in a group, discuss these reasons and functions with your colleagues. To what degree are your reasons for doing research coloured by your views about the nature of people?

Talk these things through with someone who has completed a research project. Ask them how their beliefs and values have changed (if they have) during and after the process of undertaking research. Compare your views about people with your researcher colleague's views.

CONCLUSION

Until you address some of these basic questions about people and about research you will not have clarified your motivation nor developed the ability to be critical about what you believe, think and value. Research has the interesting effect of challenging all our cherished beliefs and values. It may be a good idea to get some practice.

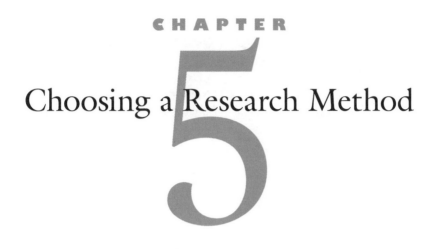

CHAPTER

Choosing a Research Method

AIMS OF THIS CHAPTER

■ To consider some of the key issues that help you to make decisions about choosing a research method.

Introduction

By now you will have clarified your research question and will be considering ways of collecting data that will help you to answer that question. The next issue is that of deciding which is the most effective means of collecting that data. Before you go ahead and collect research data, you need to be clear about the method you are going to use to collect it. In a previous chapter we noted that there are a number of theoretical or philosophical considerations to be made about what sort of research you are doing, including the debate about quantitative versus qualitative research, the question of subjectivity and objectivity, validity and reliability, sampling and so on. These issues will reappear when you come to selecting a method of data collection. By the end of this section you will be clearer about what sort of method you want to choose and how these issues are integral to choices you make about research design and data collection and analysis methods. Of course much will depend on what you want to find out.

SUGGESTED READING TO PROVIDE VARIOUS AUTHORS' DESCRIPTIONS OF RESEARCH DESIGNS

Polit, D. & Beck, C. (2010) *Essentials of Nursing Research: Appraising Evidence for Nursing Practice.* Philadelphia: Lippincott Williams & Wilkins, pp. 221–83.

Gerrish, K. & Lacey, A. (eds) (2009) *The Research Process in Nursing* (5th edn). Oxford: Blackwell Publishing, all of section 3, pp. 155–334.

Punch, K. (2005) *Introduction to Social Research: Quantitative and Qualitative Approaches* (2nd edn). London: Sage Publishing, pp. 62–84 and pp. 133–67).

The concept of research design

The term 'research design' is sometimes used to designate a particular approach to doing research. Some examples of quantitative and qualitative research designs are given below. As you read through these see if you can identify if they would most likely be employed in a quantitative or a qualitative research design or a mixture of both.

- Survey
- Experiment
- Case Study
- Ethnography
- Grounded theory
- Phenomenology
- Action Research

Survey

The survey is a systematic gathering of information from a reasonably large sample of people, events, literature, records and so forth. The purpose of a survey is usually to identify general trends or patterns in data. Examples of surveys may include:

- Nurse's attitudes to smoking;
- The number of nurses trained as enrolled nurses, at a particular hospital, during a particular period;

■ The incidence of particular illnesses in different parts of the country.

Experiment

The experiment sets out to test out a hypothesis or a theory. Experimental research tries to establish causal links between a number of factors. Examples of experimental design may include:

■ The effect of information-giving to patients on their rate of recovery from illness;

■ The effectiveness of one drug rather than another in treating a particular disorder.

Experimental research tries to prove or disprove a relationship between two or more factors using very precise measurements. Thus, in the first example above, the researcher attempts to see whether giving specific information to patients about their illness and treatment makes a difference to those patients' recovery rate from their illness. He does *not* set out to describe the *effects* of giving information – he is trying to establish a relationship between (a) the information and (b) the patient's rate of recovery measured in quite specific ways.

The experimental researcher typically uses two (sometimes more) groups of subjects in his research: the experimental group (who, in the above experiment, receive information) and the control group (who would receive no information). In both groups, the samples are selected to ensure that they are similar in all important characteristics save the one being investigated. Thus a researcher carrying out the above study would select people for both groups in terms of similarity of age, socio-economic background, weight, medical history, amount of time spent with nursing staff and so forth. The single difference between the two groups would be that one group would be given the information (the experimental group) while the other group (the control) would not be. In this way, the researcher would argue that he is ensuring that the one remaining difference (the information) did or did not affect the rate of recovery of the patients in these two groups.

The above scenario spells out the *ideal* situation. Real life is often more complicated and even a laboratory experiment can be *contaminated* in many ways. Good researchers are loath to draw firm conclusions from their findings until they have been able to reproduce very similar experimental conditions over and over again. Experiments have to be repeated several times to ensure that any differences that emerge do not just happen by chance. Even then, the question of causality is open to question and this is a debate that has raged for many years in the research literature.

Case study

The case study focus is in developing an in-depth description and understanding of the case or cases being studied by using multiple sources of data such as interviews, observations, documents and archives. The data analysis is done through description of the case and the central themes of the case. The aim of the case study approach is to 'paint a picture', to supply a description of people's thoughts, feelings and perceptions in a specific context or setting. It does not set out to prove causal relationships nor test hypotheses in the way that experimental research does. The case being studied can be a simple, easily defined unit, or it may be a complex multifaceted entity. Thus, the case could be an individual, a group, an organization, a particular incident, an event, or there are many other possibilities. A significant feature of a case study strategy, however, is that the case is bounded by space and time.

Examples, here, may be:

■ A description of how patients with multiple sclerosis cope with their disability.

■ An account of what it is like to train as a nurse during a three-year course.

Ethnography

Ethnography is a research design which seeks to describe a culture or a way of life from the point of view of the people in that culture or living that way of life. An ethnographic study requires the researcher to immerse themselves into the natural setting of the culture being studied without disturbing the setting or the participants' interactions in order to describe what is happening and how the people interpret what is happening.

An example of this type of design would be:

■ Understanding the cultural adaptations of overseas trained nurses working in a metropolitan Emergency Department.

■ Describing the health beliefs and practices of African migrants within their new migrant setting.

Grounded theory

Grounded theory research design involves the collection and analysis of data to generate a theory about the topic being studied. It is different from other designs which often seek to validate a theory, rather the grounded theory researcher starts with a clean slate in terms of explanation or understanding of the topic being studied and builds up a theory from the data collection and analysis by a process of induction.

An example of this type of study would be:

- To formulate a theory of why parents choose certain types of schools
- To identify how patients choose the general practitioner practice they are going to attend.

Phenomenology

The phenomenological approach involves seeking an understanding of a specific experience from the point of view of the individual, generally called an informant. The approach allows the researcher to learn about human consciousness and personal experience – described by the term lived experience. An important requirement of researchers who use this approach is the need to set aside (or bracket) their own assumptions and prejudices to make certain that the perspectives of the person being studied is captured in an authentic manner:

> The phenomenologist views human behavior, what people say and do, as a product of how people define their world. The task of the phenomenologist...is to capture this process of interpretation...the phenomenologist attempts to see things from other people's point of view.
>
> (Taylor & Bogdan 1984, pp. 8–9)

For example if we wanted to understand the impact of renal dialysis on a person's life so that we could provide more appropriate individualized care in the unit, we could use a phenomenological approach to undertake a research study. This would enable us to explore the individuals in the situation of 'being a dialysis patient' and to understand what the experience means to them. The purpose of phenomenology is to use the findings to provide a much richer understanding of the experience as it is lived.

Action research

Action research is a research design in which a change process and research are combined to improve something or solve problems or issues. It is a cyclic iterative process which alternates between implementing change and then using data collection and analysis processes to understand the change process and the outcomes. This cycle is repeated with the understanding gained from each cycle being used to inform the next phase of change and research. A key factor in this process is that those involved in change are part of the planning and execution of the action research cycles.

For example, if it was identified that a particular surgical ward had a much higher rate of post-operative infections than other similar wards, the ward team may decide that they wanted to improve this. Using research and reflection the team would gather data to identify the contributing factors, interventions and then decide on a strategy that would be implemented to lower the infection rate. As the strategy is implemented both the change process and the outcomes are studied to better understand the effect of the change processes on the resulting outcome. This understanding would then be used to inform the next cycle of improvement of the problem.

The list above is not exhaustive as there are other examples of research design that may be used in nursing such as historical research or philosophical research.

All of these examples of research design offer broad headings of particular approaches to research. Under each of these headings (and frequently overlapping between them) are a series of research methods of collecting and analysing research data. Just as some research designs are better suited to answer a particular research question, the same applies to data collection and analysis methods, each of which lends itself to particular designs and are unsuitable for others. The challenge is for you to ensure that the design and methods you choose to use will be suitable to gather the data required to answer your research question. It is those methods that are the subject of this and the following chapters.

Making decisions about methods

By the end of this section you will have discovered:

- Exactly what you want to find out in your project;
- What other people have found out in this field and what methods they have used to collect data.

=========================== **EXERCISE 5.1** ===========================

Aim of the exercise: To help you to state clearly what it is you want to find out in your research as a prerequisite of selecting the most appropriate method.

What to do:

1. Through a processes of brainstorming, prioritization and clarification, write *in one sentence* what your research is going to be about.

2. Having clarified your ideas, go to the library and find three studies that have already explored aspects of the field of study that interests you. From those studies answer these questions:

   ■ How did the researchers state the problem that they were researching?

   ■ In what ways were the problems stated in those projects similar to and different to your own?

   ■ What methods of data collection did they use?

   ■ Could any of the data collection methods used be suitable for your project? If so why, if not why not?

   ■ In what ways will your research project clarify the field or add to the body of knowledge?

   ■ Why are you choosing *this* problem?

Discuss your research intention and the answers to the above questions with colleagues and with a supervisor. Has the exercise made you modify your original research statement in any way or has it confirmed your need to pursue that line of inquiry?

Validity and reliability

Other issues that you need to consider concern validity and reliability. Validity and reliability are words you will encounter repeatedly in your reading about research. They tend to be associated with the notion of measurement in research and standards of reliability and validity need to be demonstrated if others are to have confidence in our research findings. The concepts of validity and reliability are important because they are central to whether the research findings can be trusted.

Stated simply, validity refers to whether an instrument measures what it sets out to measure. Here is an example. If you wanted to check a person's body temperature you would probably use a clinical thermometer filled with mercury because you know this instrument will provide a valid (*accurate/truthful*) measure of a person's temperature – 37°C. We also know that if the person has an infection that their body temperature will change and this will be indicated on the thermometer.

Reliability refers to whether or not a measuring instrument works *consistently* in producing similar results in similar situations. The clinical thermometer is a reliable measuring instrument as it provides consistent results – assuming practitioners use it in the same way with people in their care. It is fit for the purpose described. It would not however be a useful measuring instrument if we needed to take the temperature of an African elephant. Instead this may require the elephant to ingest a temperature sensor which can be retrieved later from the elephant's dung. Incidentally an elephant's temperature tends to be lower than humans (about 36.5°C).

The measurement of physical things tends to be relatively straightforward. However when we try to measure human qualities it can be very tricky – for example are female nurses more 'caring' than male nurses? The issues of validity and reliability become much more difficult when we try to develop specific measures of personality or attitude. Is it possible for example to develop a reliable and valid attitudinal measure of 'caring' which is supposed to be a core construct for most of the helping professions? Would a high score on such a scale indicate a higher quality of care experienced by patients and clients? In a neat summary of the validity and reliability Lacey writes:

> A study to assess the health effects of air pollution in a community would not be valid if it simply collected people's views about air quality, without measuring actual levels of disease or even mortality rates...(and)...A set of weighing scales that give a person's weight as 52kg at 10:00am and 55kg at 10:05 could not be said to be reliable.
>
> (Lacey 2006, pp. 28–9)

Although there is some debate about the terms validity and reliability being applied to qualitative research because they are generally associated with the measurement in quantitative terms, the requirements of a rigorous process to ensure the quality and trustworthiness of the research remains the same whether it is a quantitative or qualitative research project. Terms such as credibility, transferability, dependability, trustworthiness and objectivity are more generally used in qualitative research to describe the level of rigour displayed in the research process. The onus is on the researcher to demonstrate this when writing up the project.

An engaging story

The famous little story of the blind men and the elephant can be a very helpful stimulus for a discussion about validity and reliability in the classroom and serve as an important reminder to researchers about the dangers of focussing on complex things from a single, limited perspective.

The Blind Men and the Elephant

It was six men of Hindostan,
To learning much inclined,

Who went to see the elephant,
(Though all of them were blind);
That each by observation
Might satisfy his mind.
The first approached the elephant,
And happening to fall
Against his broad and sturdy side,
At once began to bawl,
"Bless me, it seems the elephant
Is very like a wall."
The second, feeling of his tusk,
Cried, "Ho! What have we here
So very round and smooth and sharp?
To me 'tis mighty clear
This wonder of an elephant
Is very like a spear."
The third approached the animal,
And happening to take
The squirming trunk with his hand,
Then boldly up and spake;
"I see" quoth he, "the elephant
Is very like a snake."
The fourth stretched out his eager hand
And felt about the knee,
"What most this mighty beast is like
Is mighty plain," quoth he;
"Tis clear enough the elephant
Is very like a tree."
The fifth who chanced to touch the ear
Said, "Even the blindest man
Can tell what this resembles most;
Deny the fact who can,
This marvel of an elephant
Is very like a fan."
The sixth no sooner had begun
About the beast to grope
Than, seizing on the swinging tail
That fell within his scope,
"I see," cried he, "the elephant
Is very like a rope."
And so these men of Hindostan
Disputed loud and long,
Each of his own opinion
Exceeding stiff and strong,
Though each was partly in the right,
And all were in the wrong!
        John Godfrey Saxe (1816–87)

The requirements for validity and reliability have to be addressed differently when using quantitative and qualitative approaches to research. Moreover the extent to which these must be covered will depend on the nature of the project. We recommend that you explore some of the following references on issues of validity and reliability. Validity and reliability are so central to research that they will crop up in nearly all books that you read about research.

SUGGESTED READING

This should include the following:

Creswell, J. (2007) *Qualitative Inquiry & Research Design: Choosing Among Five Approaches* (2nd edn). California: Sage Publications, pp. 202–13.

Robson, C. (2002) *Real World Research: A Resource for Social Scientists and Practitioner-Researchers* (2nd edn). Blackwell, Oxford, pp. 101–10.

Before we actually get down to the process of choosing a data collection and analysis method there is one further area of information that you must consider and that is how will you choose the participants from whom you will collect the data. Choosing the most appropriate sampling method to find the information needed to address your research question is also crucial to ensuring that at the end of your project you have credible results that will stand the test of acceptability by peers.

Sampling methods

The purpose of research is usually to explore various themes and trends throughout a certain population of people (e.g. all the nurses in the United Kingdom or all the nurses working in medical wards in a group of hospitals). It is usually impractical to attempt to collect data from every member of that population. Therefore, it is necessary to choose a sample from that population. A sample is a group of people from a larger population (although a sample may also be a collection of records, a number of observations and so on). It is usual to try to select a sample of people that is representative of the larger group. There are various ways of selecting a sample which will be influenced by some of the following:

- The design of the study – depth or breadth approach

- The type of information needed – quantitative or qualitative or both
- The timeframe and resources available to you
- Your access to respondents/cases/settings
- The ethical issues elicited by the study
- The associated costs

Fortunately there are several different types of sampling techniques available which take account of the various designs and methods and help to ensure that projects can be completed in an efficient and rigorous manner. These include the following:

- Simple random sampling – selection of the sample from the study population at random
- Stratified random sampling – dividing the study population into groups by certain characteristics (e.g. males, females) and then random sampling within each of the groups
- Cluster sampling – dividing the study population into clusters with a range of characteristics and then sampling from within the clusters
- Quota sampling – quotas for specific characteristics or categories are identified and the sample is collected from these categories until the quota is reached.
- Convenience sampling – selects the most convenient sample readily available
- Purposive sampling – sample chosen on the basis of judgement that they will have information about the topic being studied
- Snowball sampling – sample is selected by referral from other participants
- Strategic informant sampling – sample of expert informants

The first four of these sampling techniques tend to be associated with large-scale survey designs focusing on breadth and using quantitative analysis. The remainder tend to be associated with more qualitative in-depth designs focussing on depth like case studies and ethnographies.

You may find the following references useful when considering how to select a sample for a quantitative and /or a qualitative study:

SUGGESTED READING

Coyne, I. (1997) Sampling in qualitative research. Purposeful and theoretical sampling; merging or clear boundaries? *Journal of Advanced Nursing* 26: 623–30.

Hart, M. (2007) Birthing a research project: sampling. *International Journal of Childbirth Education* 22(2): 31–4.

http://www.socialresearchmethods.net/kb/sampling.php

http://www.statpac.com/surveys/sampling.htm

Sheu, S., Wei, I., Chen, C. Yu, S. & Tang, F. (2009) Using snowball sampling method with nurses to understand medication and administration errors. *Journal of Clinical Nursing* 18(4): 559–69.

Shields, L. (2008) Sampling in quantitative research. *Paediatric Nursing* 20(5): 37.

The sample that you require for your study will be determined to a large degree by what you are researching, what methods you are using, and the time you have available. As you become more familiar with the literature covering your particular area of interest, the research designs, methods and samples used, this will help clarify your thinking and decision-making about your project.

CONCLUSION

You should now be clearer about how you want to conduct your research project and how this fits within the context of earlier studies. Adopting a general research design will give you a broad template for thinking about how you might gather information that will address the issues or questions you have. It also provides some general indicators about the sorts of sampling that might be appropriate and how the general issues of validity and reliability might be considered. In the following chapters we will consider more closely the specific data collection and analysis options available to you.

CHAPTER

Methods of Collecting Data

6

AIMS OF THIS CHAPTER

- To explore methods of data collection;

- To identify the strengths and limitations of each method;

- To enable you to consider the usefulness or otherwise of each of these methods for your own research project.

Introduction

In the last chapter we suggested ways that you might make decisions about how to collect data for your project. In this chapter we look at specific data collection methods. You may already have decided what methods you are likely to use but it will be useful to read this chapter and do the exercises. This way you will familiarize yourself with other methods and you may find that you want to change your data collection method, either slightly or radically. If not, you will confirm that your original decision was right.

This chapter is in two parts. The first deals with those methods that are very well established in the research field. In the second part of the chapter we will consider some other ways of collecting data that are not used as often in nursing research but that you may find suits your particular project.

Part one: Frequently used data collection methods

Traditional ways of finding out things have tended to be:

- Talking to people;

- Asking people to answer questions;

- Doing experiments;

- Watching how things happen, that is, how people interact or do things

The common terms to describe these research activities are:

- Interviews

- Questionnaires

- Experiments

- Observation.

Interviews

Interviews can be undertaken with any number of people but each person is usually interviewed separately. There are research projects that are better suited to interviewing groups of people together. A group interview is called a focus group and is becoming more widely used in nursing research. Before you choose interviews as a data collection method you will need to know the following:

- What a structured interview is;

- The difference between a structured interview, semi-structured and an unstructured interview;

- The advantages and limitations of choosing to interview groups of people;

- How to analyse interviews;

- The limitations of the use of interviews.

Structured interviews

A structured interview uses an *interview schedule* which, in its strongest form, is like a *questionnaire*. The researcher uses a list of set questions which is asked of every person who is interviewed. The interview schedule is developed and piloted well before the main interviews take place and is designed to cover everything that the researcher wants to find out from the respondents. One of the advantages of this approach is that it allows the researcher to organize and analyse the findings relatively easily. After the interviews, all the responses to the first question can be drawn together, all the responses to the second and so on. On the other hand, the structured interview allows no scope for *in-depth* interviewing. The interviewer cannot follow up subsequent questions that occur to her/him after the interview, nor can he or she follow 'hunches' and ask the respondent to elaborate on particular issues during the interview. This is particularly important if the researcher also wants to find out *why* people feel the way they do: the structured interview tends not to access this sort of information.

The structured interview cannot, by its design, cope with the spontaneous responses that people make nor the off-the-cuff impressions that respondents may want to offer. On the other hand, it can offer an economical way of gathering a lot of useful information quickly. The *depth* of the interview is largely determined by the *nature of the research questions* and the *level of understanding required by the researcher.*

Semi-structured interviews

An alternative to the completely structured interview is the *semi-structured* one. In the semi-structured interview, the researcher has a number of fixed questions prepared beforehand but scope is built in to ask *subsequent* questions, should the need arise. This breaks up the strict format of the structured approach and can yield 'richer' data. As well as obtaining *quantitative* data (from the structured part of the interview) the researcher also obtains more *qualitative* data (in the form of opinions, explanations and personal accounts). On the other hand, the data that arise out of these interviews can be more difficult to analyse because of the fact that the structure is not fixed and there will be a variety of responses.

Unstructured interviews

The unstructured interview takes a very different approach to data collection. Usually, the researcher has some idea of the area on which they want to focus the interview but, after that, the researcher remains open to whatever the respondent wants to say about that area of study. In this style of interviewing, the *respondent* has much more control over how the interview proceeds. The researcher can have little idea, beforehand, what *sort* of interview he or she will be conducting, nor can they know in advance what sorts of things the respondent will talk about. The net result of all this is that the researcher is likely to be faced with a wide range of different sorts of personal accounts that require analysis.

Necessarily, the analysis of unstructured interviews is different to the analysis of structured ones. Various analysis methods have been devised to cope with the varied nature of the information gleaned from unstructured interviews. Some of these include the following:

- Content analysis
- Phenomenological analysis
- Grounded theory analysis
- Ethnographic analysis.

If you are thinking about using the unstructured approach to interviews, you *must* know, beforehand, how you will analyse the interview transcripts. This is, of course, true, of *all* data collection methods: you *must* know, before you collect your data, how you will analyse it.

The following points should be borne in mind when using unstructured interviews:

- They are very time consuming: an interview may last half and hour or it may run for a number of hours.

- They should be taped – you cannot expect to remember the details of what was said in an interview if you rely on taking notes.

- The tapes should be transcribed. That is to say that all the words that are spoken by both the interviewer and the respondent should be written or typed out afterwards. This task can be made easier with the help of specialist software such as Leximancer (https://leximancer. thecustomerinsightportal.com/). There is some debate about whether or not this *always* has to happen. Some writers have suggested that you can work directly from the tapes. We suggest that you only use this approach once you have had considerable experience of working with unstructured interview.

- Whatever method of analysis you use, you must be clear about both the theoretical and *procedural* approaches that are to be adopted. Phenomenological and grounded theory approaches, for example, are based on highly complex philosophical ideas about the nature of knowledge and about ways of doing research. If you want to use these approaches, you need to know about these things. If not, you will be safer using a form of simple *content analysis*. There has been a tendency, in recent years, for some nurse researchers to use terms such as 'phenomenological' and 'hermeneutic' in fairly loose ways, and others have claimed that their studies involved 'modified grounded theory'. Theoretical clarity is essential in these matters – particularly in the qualitative field.

Focus groups

Interviewing people in groups is useful when the researcher is seeking an in-depth understanding of the views of a selected group on an issue or topic. It is useful when the researcher wants to know not only what the group thinks about certain things, but also why and the differing views that may be held by people within the group. The interview can use structured, semi-structured or a completely unstructured interview format. The advantages of using focus groups is that they are a quick and flexible way of gathering a variety of opinions and the group setting can stimulate discussions and views that a one-on-one interview may not. The disadvantage of focus groups is that they require considerable preparation and the researcher has to be skilled in the techniques facilitating group discussion. It may be difficult to stop dominant people 'taking over' the discussion and those who may hold contrary opinions to the majority may not feel comfortable to put these forward. It is useful when conducting a focus group to have two people involved – one to moderate the group and the other to observe. The interviewer also needs to be aware of their own biases and ensure that they do not control the responses within the group.

SUGGESTED FURTHER READING

Berg, B. L. (2008) *Qualitative Research Methods for the Social Sciences* (7th edn). Boston, MA: Allyn & Bacon (a wide range of chapters covering interviewing, focus groups and content analysis presented in an easy to read format).

Neuendorf, K. (2002) *The Content Analysis Guidebook*. California: Sage Publications, pp. 1–22.

Graneheim, U. H. & Lundman, B. (2004) Qualitative content analysis in nursing research: Concepts, procedures and measures to achieve trustworthiness. *Nurse Education Today* 24(2): 105–12.

http://qualitativeresearch.ratcliffs.net/5.htm

Goodman, C. & Evans, C. (2006) Using focus groups. In K. Gerrish & A. Lacey (eds) *The Research Process in Nursing*. Oxford: Blackwell Publishing, pp. 352–66.

Marshall, M., Carter, B., Rose, K. & Brotherton, A. (2009) Living with type 1 diabetes: Perspectives of children and their parents. *Journal of Clinical Nursing* 18(12): 1703–10.

Newell, R. & Burnard, P. (2010a) *Research for Evidence-Based Practice* (2nd edn). Oxford: Blackwell, pp. 57–117.

Rejeh, N., Ahmadi, F., Mohammadi, E., Kazemnejad, A. & Anoosheh, M. (2009) Nurses' experiences and perceptions of influencing barriers to postoperative pain management. *Scandinavian Journal of Caring Sciences* 23(2): 274–81.

Robson, C. (2002) *Real World Research: A Resource for Social Scientists and Practitioner-Researchers* (2nd edn). Oxford: Wiley-Blackwell, pp. 269–91.

Usher, K., Baker, J. A., Holmes, C. & Stocks, B. (2009) Clinical decision-making for 'as needed' medications in mental health care. *Journal of Advanced Nursing* 65(5): 981–91.

EXERCISE 6.1

Aim of the exercise: To explore the use of the unstructured interview.

What to do: Ask a friend to give you ten minutes of their time. In those ten minutes and without prior preparation, ask them to tell you about their work. Encourage the flow of conversation by asking any questions that come to mind and which have a bearing on the topic. Make notes about your colleague's responses or make a tape recording of the interview. If you can, repeat the process with one other friend.

Evaluation: When you have completed the interview(s), ask yourself the following questions about the data you have in front of you:

- Does it represent a detailed account of the colleague's work?
- Did the conversation 'flow' in an orderly manner and have a beginning, a middle and an end?
- What did I learn about the person's experience of their work?
- How much did I talk during the interview?
- To what degree did I influence the sort of answers that the colleague offered?
- What are some of the pros and cons of simply asking people to talk about their work or aspects of their lives?
- If two people were interviewed, was the content of both interviews similar in depth and breadth?
- Could I have collected the data more effectively?

■ How did the use of unstructured interviews contribute to my skills as a researcher?

■ How could the use of unstructured interviews help me to refine my research questions?

■ What sort of problems will I have in analysing these data?

You have conducted an unstructured interview. Such an approach may be useful in certain circumstances and we will return to this issue further on in this chapter. The structured interview offers alternative method of collecting information about a topic. As you work through the next exercise, consider the advantages and disadvantages of the structured approach to interviewing. The structured interview is distinguished by at least the following criteria:

■ There are a limited number of questions.

■ These questions have a specified number of possible answers.

■ The answers are easier to quantify than the answers identified by the unstructured approach.

■ The researcher specifies the questions to be asked.

EXERCISE 6.2

Aim of the exercise: To devise a short structured interview schedule and to use this as a basis for carrying out an interview.

What to do: Write out ten questions that you would like to ask someone about their job (see the section headed 'Open and closed questions', about different sorts of questions). Then ask those questions of your colleague and note down their answers. If possible, repeat the process with one or more colleagues.

Evaluation: Look at the responses that you elicited from your colleague(s) and ask yourself the following questions:

■ Did I find out what I wanted to find out?

■ Did my questions elicit the sort of answers that I anticipated that they would?

■ How will I analyse the answers that I was offered?

■ How could I improve my interview schedule?

If you can, discuss your questions and your colleague(s) responses with someone who has used a structure interview approach in his own research. Develop with your colleagues a list of the pros and cons of the unstructured and structured approaches to interviewing. Discuss when the unstructured and the structured approaches may be used to advantage.

Interviews used in research need not be of an entirely unstructured or an entirely structured nature. Many research reports combine both styles to very good effect. Now read some of the following sources about interviewing:

Price, B. (2002) Laddered questions and qualitative data research inter-views. *Journal of Advanced Nursing* 37: 273–81.

Rubin, H. J. & Rubin, I. S. (2005) *Qualitative Interviewing: The Art of Hearing Data* (2nd edn). Thousand Oaks, CA: Sage.

Open and closed questions

There are two types of questions. Closed questions are those that elicit a restricted range of answers (in extreme, these answers may be 'yes' or 'no'). In some cases, the interviewer offers the respondent the range of possible answers. Examples of closed questions are:

- Do you smoke? Yes/ No
- How satisfied are you with your present state of health? Very satis-fied/ Satisfied/ Uncertain/Dissatisfied/Very satisfied

Open questions are those that elicit answers that the interviewer cannot anticipate and are usually lengthier and more divergent than the answers to closed questions. Open questions usually begin with the words: what, why, where or how? Examples of open questions are:

- What are your views on smoking?
- Why are you dissatisfied with your health?

Both closed and open questions can be used in research interviews. Methods of analysing the data obtained from the two types of ques-tion may differ. Structured interviews that use closed questions may be analysed *quantitatively*. Unstructured interviews that use open ques-tions may be analysed *qualitatively*. In between these two extremes are semi-structured interviews that may combine open and closed questions about the same topic. These semi-structured interviews may be analysed using both quantitative and/or qualitative methods.

Questionnaires

Simply stated, the questionnaire differs from the structured interview only by the degree of personal involvement on the part of the researcher at the point of data collection.

You will need to know the following:

■ What a questionnaire is;

■ What types of questionnaire there are;

■ What are the advantages and disadvantages of questionnaires?

Two types of questionnaire

There are at least two major types of questionnaires: those that attempt to measure the structure and strength of attitudes and those that gather information about things. The attitudinal questionnaire consists of a series of questions that check people's opinions about events, situations, people and/ or concepts. An attitudinal questionnaire might be used to identify people's attitudes towards mentally ill people being looked after in the community or patients' satisfaction levels with regard to their care in hospital. Attitudinal questions tend to focus on how people *think, feel* or *behave* with regard to the topic under consideration. Attitudinal questionnaires can often result in an overall *score*. This scoring mechanism usually operates on the basis that a *low* score relates to a *negative* attitude while a *high* score relates to a *positive* attitude.

A common method of collecting attitudinal data from a question-naire is the inclusion of *Likert-type* items (named after the psychologist, Rene Likert). Figure 6.1 shows an example of such an item. Study the characteristics of the scale, try to do a little reading around the use of Likert scales (see 'Suggested further reading', below).

Questionnaires that gather information about things do just that: they ask the respondent to report particular and specific information by ticking boxes or by answering specific questions – often in a 'yes/ no' format. These sorts of questionnaires cannot be *scored*, but these can be counted and frequencies and proportions can be determined. The information that is gathered from them can be illustrated in a series of tables, bar graphs and pie charts to highlight trends and patterns in the data. An example of an information-seeking questionnaire might be one that asks respondents about their nurse education, previous work experience and current job. The information that was gleaned from such

	Strongly agree	Agree	Undecided	Disagree	Strongly disagree	Please leave blank
I get paid enough for the job I do						

Figure 6.1 Example of *Likert-type* data collection questionnaire

a questionnaire might include the respondents' ages, sex, qualifications, training experiences and so forth.

Some questionnaires combine *both* forms of information gathering. It is important, however, to be clear about *which* questions are of an 'attitudinal' type and which are of an 'information gathering' type. This combination technique can allow the researcher to explore relationships (or lack of them) between concrete information and views and opinions. The researcher might, for example, want to explore whether there were differences in perceptions about mentally ill people between mental health nurses and *general* nurses. To do this, the researcher would have to collect some information about the nurses' background *as well* as asking them about their attitudes.

SUGGESTED FURTHER READING

Anthonak, R. F. and Livneh, H. (1988) *The Measurement of Attitudes Towards People with Disabilities: Methods, Psychometrics and Scales.* Springfield, IL: Charles C. Thomas (has lots of examples of Likert and other scales).

Fraser, L. & Lawley, M. (2000) *Questionnaire Design & Administration: A Practical Guide.* Brisbane, Australia: John Wiley & Sons (a really practical book on all aspects of the art of asking questions in different formats).

Sommer, B. and Sommer, R. (2002) *A Practical Guide to Behavioural Research: Tools and Techniques* (5th edn). Oxford: Oxford University Press (a really good overview of the research process and data collection in an easy to read format with interesting examples).

Questionnaire construction

Designing questionnaires is not easy. Oppenheim, in the preface to his classic book on questionnaire design, had this to say:

> The world is full of well-meaning people who believe that anyone who can write plain English and has a modicum of common sense can produce a good questionnaire. This book is not for them.
>
> (Oppenheim 1992, preface)

As a rule, if there is a ready-made questionnaire (measure, instrument, scale) to hand, that has been properly tested for validity and reliability, which you do not have to modify, then you are best advised to use that.

If you *have* or want to design a questionnaire, May (1993) suggests the following stages:

1. What is the aim of the research?

2. What information is required to fulfil these aims?

3. Undertake preliminary reading around the topic and initial field-work.

4. What type of questionnaire will be used and how will the sample be derived?

5. Consider the most appropriate questions to ask, which will depend upon the aims of the research, the target group and the time and resources at your disposal.

6. Construct a first draft, taking into account that pre-coded questions are easier to analyse and the order of question is the best social-psychological sequence.

7. Pilot the questionnaire and elicit the opinions of the sub-sample, gain critical but supportive comments from those familiar with the design and analysis of questionnaires.

8. Edit the questionnaire to check on form, content and sequence of questions; make sure the questionnaire is neatly typed; all instructions and coding are clear; and filter questions, if any, are understandable.

9. Administer the questionnaire, noting the dynamics for the interviews and comments of the interviewers (if used).

10. Analyse the questionnaire drawing upon statistical techniques.

If you do decide to develop a questionnaire yourself, you would be well advised to consult a good source:

SUGGESTED READING

Alreck, P. L. & Settle, R. B. (2004) *The Survey Research Handbook* (3rd edn). Columbus, OH: McGraw-Hill, pp. 89–130.

Meadows, K. A. (2003) So you want to do research? 5: Questionnaire design. *British Journal of Community Nursing* 8(12): 562–70.

Krosnic, J. & Presser, S. (2010) Questions and questionnaire design. In J. Wright & Marsden (eds), *Handbook of Survey Research* (2nd edn). San Diego, CA, Elsevier, pp. 263–315.

Lumsden, J. (2007) Online questionnaire design. In R. Reynolds & R. Woods (eds) *Handbook of Research on Electronic Survey Measurement*, pp. 44–64. London: Idea Group Reference.

Oppenheim, A. N. (1992) *Questionnaire Design, Interviewing and Attitude Measurement* (2nd edn). London: Pinter (a classic that is still very useful and easy to read).

EXERCISE 6.3

Aim of the exercise: To become familiar with various types of questionnaires.

What to do: Sit down and draw up a short questionnaire of six questions. The questions should be designed to answer one of the following research questions:

- Is nursing stressful?
- Are some nurses more assertive than others?
- Do nurses use a nursing model in their practice?

Do no prior reading before attempting this part of the exercise.

When you have written your six questions, go to the library and find the following books.

Fraser, L. & Lawley, M. (2000) *Questionnaire Design & Administration: A Practical Guide*. Brisbane, Australia: John Wiley & Sons.

Bradburn, N. M., Sudman, S. & Wansink, B. (2004) *Asking Questions: The Definitive to Questionnaire Design for Market Research, Political Polls, and Social and Health Questionnaires*. San Francisco: Jossey Bass.

Read the sections on questionnaires and answer the following questions:

- What is a questionnaire?
- What is a questionnaire for?
- What distinguishes a questionnaire from an interview?
- How may questionnaire data be analysed?
- What principles go into the production of questionnaires?

Now read your own questions and see to what degree they need to be modified. Then try to modify them in the light of your reading.

Try out your modified questionnaire on a friend. Ask her to act as 'devil's advocate' and raise any objections she may have about the construction of your short questionnaire. Try, also, to show the questionnaire to a lecturer or to someone with research experience and ask their opinion of your work.

Advantages and disadvantages of questionnaires

Advantages

- Questionnaires offer a straightforward way of collecting data, quickly and efficiently.
- They are cheap to use.
- They enable the researcher to collect information anonymously.
- They are usually easy to analyse.
- Large batches of data can be collected with them.

Disadvantages

- The researcher has no personal contact with the respondent.
- They can be difficult to construct.
- They involve 'forced choice' of response from the respondent.

Try to add to both of these lists, from your reading on the topic.

Experiments

Experiments are systematic attempts to test out a theory (usually stated in the form of a hypothesis). Experimental research tries to identify causal relationships between variables, and tries to establish 'laws'. It is not anticipated that many nurses coming fresh to research will be planning experimental studies. It is useful, however, to be able to read experimental research studies both for their content and to be critical of them.

You will need to know the following:

- What a hypothesis is;
- Some of the terms associated with data collection and experimental research;
- How to become critical of experimental research reports.

═══════════════ **EXERCISE 6.4** ═══════════════

Aim of the exercise: To explore some of the terms used in experimental research.

Stage one

Exploring the terms hypothesis and null hypothesis.

What to do: Go to the library and find the following books or any other general research book. Look up the word hypothesis and read the relevant sections:

Gerrish, K. & Lacey, A. (eds) (2006) *The Research Process in Nursing* (5th edn). Oxford: Blackwell.

Newell, R. & Burnard, P. (2010a) *Research for Evidence-Based Practice* (2nd edn). Oxford: Blackwell.

Robson, C. (2002) *Real World Research: A Resource for Social Scientists and Practitioner-Researchers* (2nd edn). Oxford: Wiley-Blackwell.

Evaluation: Ask yourself the following questions:

■ What is a hypothesis?

■ What is a null hypothesis?

■ How do you use a hypothesis?

■ What is the difference between a hypothesis and an assumption?

■ What does the term 'variable' mean?

Now talk to your colleagues or lecturer about the concept of a hypothesis.

Stage two

Using the books from stage one of this exercise, or any other general research book, devise definitions for the following terms. Make notes of your definitions.

■ Control group

■ Experimental group

■ Statistical significance

■ Sampling

■ Confounding variables

■ Population

■ Intervention

■ Outcome

■ Testing effects

- Temporal effects
- Regression to the mean
- Randomization
- Hawthorne effect

Now read the following two research reports and note how these terms are used. In coming to terms with the concepts involved in the use of these words, you are beginning to get to grips with the concepts involved in doing experimental work. As you read these reports, try to evaluate the degree to which the writers have addressed problems presented by these concepts.

Reynolds, T., Russell, L., Deeth, M., Jones, H. & Birchall, L. (2004) A randomised controlled trial comparing Drawtex with standard dressings for exuding wounds. *Journal of Wound Care* 13(2): 71–4.

Aranda, S., Schofield, P., Weih, L., Milne, D., Yates, P. & Faulkner, R. (2006) Meeting the support and information needs of women with advanced breast cancer: A randomised controlled trial. *The British Journal of Cancer* 95(6): 667.

Edwards, H., Courtney, M., Finlayson, K., Shuter, P. & Lindsay, E. (2009) A randomized controlled trial of a community nursing intervention: Improved quality of life and healing for clients with chronic leg ulcers. *Journal of Clinical Nursing* 18(11): 1541–9.

Discuss the above terms with friends and with a lecturer and make sure that you are clear about their use.

Observation

By the end of this section, you will have discovered:

- What sort of information is being sought through observation;
- Some of the problems associated with observation;
- What types of observational methods can be used.

EXERCISE 6.5

Aim of the exercise: To explore problems and practical issues associated with observation.

What to do:

Stage one

Go to somewhere crowded or busy (e.g. a bus station, an outpatients department, a staff cafeteria). Sit and observe people for about ten minutes. Make notes about your observations.

Now consider the following questions:

- What sort of things did you observe?
- How did you decide on what to observe and what to ignore?
- How did you make notes on what you observed?
- Did you try to interpret what people were doing and why they were doing it?
- Did anyone notice you and ask what you were doing?

In considering these issues, you are beginning to appreciate the difficulties that all researchers face when trying to decide on how to collect data by means of observation. Some researchers have found it useful to use a system for recording what they see.

Stage two

First, identify in your own mind what it is you want to observe when you go to the crowded place, identified above. You might, for instance, be interested in how many people get on a particular bus when it stops at a bus station, or you might want to observe how many people choose salad as a meal in the staff cafe. What you can never do is observe everything that is going on in any given situation. You must decide what is important for your project. You must also try to refrain from interpreting what you see. You are not there to make assumptions about people's behaviour, you are there to observe and record. At a later stage, you may want to ask people why they did things but that comes later.

To aid your observation, draw up a simple checklist or grid to help you record what you see. Now go back to the crowded place for a further ten minutes, use your checklist, and observe again.

Now ask yourself the following questions:

- Was the second stage of the exercise easier or more difficult than the first?
- In what ways did your checklist help or hinder you?
- Did your checklist work?

In these two activities, you have explored some of the problems associated with observation in research. Now read the following to clarify further how observational methods may be used to collect research data. Read, too, the section on 'Aspects of observation in research'.

Watson, H. & White, R. (2006) Using observation. In K. Gerrish & A. Lacey (eds) *The Research Process in Nursing.* Oxford: Blackwell Publishing, pp. 383–98.

Polit, D. & Beck, C. (2010) *Essentials of Nursing Research: Appraising Evidence for Nursing Practice.* Philadelphia: Lippincott Williams & Wilkins, pp. 178–84, 351–9.

Aspects of observation in research

Two types of observational method

1. *Non-Participant Observation*: Here, the researcher enters a social setting as an observer and sits and records examples of behaviour or action that he is researching. He does not attempt to influence the situation that he is in and does not attempt to stop anything from happening. On the other hand, of course, the very presence of the researcher may change what is happening. This is called the 'Hawthorne Effect'.

2. *Participant Observation*: Here, the researcher enters a social situation and works alongside the people in that situation, thus fulfilling a dual role (a) as a worker and (b) as an observer.

You may want to consider the pros and cons of these two approaches, whether there are ethical problems with either approach, or the appropriateness of either in answering a particular research question.

Sommer and Sommer (2002) offer the following list of steps for systematic observation:

1. Specify the question(s) of interest (reason for doing the study).

2. Do casual observation, distinguishing between observation (the actual behaviour seen) and inference (interpretation, what you think it means).

3. Are the observational categories clearly described?

4. Design the measurement instruments (i.e. checklists, categories, coding systems, etc.).

5. Is the study designed so that it will be *valid* (i.e. does it measure what it is supposed to measure and have some generalizability)?

6. Train observers in the use of the instruments.

7. Do a pilot test.

   a. Test the actual observation procedure.

   b. Check reliability of the categories using at least two independent observers.

8. Review procedure and instruments in the light of the pilot test results. If substantial changes are made, run another pilot test.

9. Collect data.

10. Compile, analyse and interpret results.

Part two: Other data collection methods

In part one we considered four methods of collecting data: interviews, questionnaires, experiments and observation. We noted that these were perhaps the most frequently used methods in many social science research projects, including those carried out in nursing. In part two we examine some other methods that you may want to consider for your project or which you may come across in your search and examination of the literature and previous research. As we have noted, there is no right or wrong way of collecting data. Different projects, different research questions and different levels of experience will influence the decision to choose one method rather than another. Appropriate choice of method is the key to success in research and arguably it is useful to have an informed awareness of a wide range of such methods.

The methods we consider in part two are:

- use of existing records
- repertory grid technique
- critical incident technique
- multiple sorting technique
- use of existing scales, inventories, tests and assessment tools
- delphi method

This is not an exhaustive list of all possible data collection techniques and you are advised to be on the look out for other methods not covered in this book. Our aim here is to give you a flavour of some other ways of approaching your project.

SUGGESTED READING

This should include the following:

Boswell, C. & Cannon, S. (2007) *Introduction to Nursing Research: Incorporating Evidence-Based Practice*. Sudbury, MA: Jones and Bartlett, pp. 217–48.

Minichiello, V., Sullivan, G., Greenwood, K. & Axford, R. (eds) (2004) *Handbook for Research Methods for Nursing and Health Sciences*. Frenchs Forest, NSW: Prentice-Hall, pp. 297–449.

Use of existing records

By the end of this section you will have discovered:

- What sort of records can be used in a research project;
- How to gain access to records;
- How to use records in research.

Sources of existing data

Doing research is not always about collecting new data. Sometimes we can begin an important project by examining data that is readily available. It can be extremely informative to explore existing datasets. These can often lead to researchers asking new and important questions, or can shed light on 'real world' problems, without the need to design and execute large-scale studies. Exploring existing data can lead to changes in practice grounded in evidence. In some instances there are many datasets sitting waiting to be re-examined and many are published routinely to profile the delivery of services. Here are some of the sources of such datasets:

- Lists of accidents and incidents occurring in clinical areas
- In psychiatric units, records of disturbed behaviour and of seclusion
- Existing datasets collected by colleagues and friends during other research projects

- Rosters and workload patterns and other management records
- Patterns of admission and discharge
- Patient or client outcome measures
- Rates of unit-acquired infections
- Medication errors
- Important social and health trends are published regularly – see
    - http://www.sirc.org/,
    - http://www.aihw.gov.au/subjectareas.cfm

=========================== **EXERCISE 6.6** ===========================

Aim of the exercise: To explore the use of collecting data from a set of existing records.

What to do: Go to the following website: http://www.aihw.gov.au/publications/index.cfm/title/10677#detailed_tables

Review the types of information that are contained in these records. For example, characteristics of health and community services workers

- Industry of health and community services workers
- Demographics of workers
- Indigenous health and community services workers
- Hours worked
- Highest qualification

Devise a simple method of collecting *some* of that information onto one sheet. Then look through the data that you have collected and see if any particular *patterns* occur within those data. For example if you are looking at the demographic characteristics:

- How many indigenous people were employed in health and community services occupations in 2006?
- Of these how many indigenous people were employed in the Indigenous community services workforce in 2006?
- Has there been a change in the number of indigenous people employed in health and community workforce between 2001 and 2006?

Gradually, you will be able to develop a partial picture from the data that will tell you a considerable amount about the characteristics of the health workforce in 2006 in Australia. This picture will be considerably more detailed *after* you have filtered out certain trends and patterns than was the case before you sat down with the records.

This approach to working with records can lead you to ask other questions about the topic that you are interested in and can point your research in other, more useful, directions that may not have been at first apparent.

Repertory grid technique

By the end of this section you will have discovered:

- Whether Kelly's repertory grid technique may be usefully considered for your own research project.

Personal construct theory and repertory grids

The repertory grid technique is based on Kelly's (1955) personal construct theory. In its simplest form it seeks to identify the characteristics that an individual looks for in other people and in the world around him. These characteristics, Kelly calls 'constructs' and he argues that they are usually bipolar or two-sided in nature. Thus the person who sees some people as 'caring' by nature, will tend to compare those people to others that they see as being 'uncaring'. Kelly also argued that each person's set of ways of seeing other things or people (her 'constructs'), varied from person to person.

Kelly used the word 'element' to describe events, things, people that are being viewed by the person through her construct system. Thus, it is possible to consider three elements: (a) a friend, (b) a doctor and (c) a nurse. It is then possible to consider in what ways *two* of those elements are similar and different from the third. For example, you may consider that the doctor and the nurse are both *professionals* and the friend is *not professional*. Alternatively, you may consider that the nurse and the friend are both *approachable* and the doctor is *distant*. In these examples, then, the friend, doctor and nurse are *elements* and the descriptions *professional–not professional* and *approachable–distant* are both bipolar *constructs*.

This approach to identifying people's characteristic ways of viewing people and the world around them can be exploited for the purposes of research. The approach may be used to find out how a group of nurses perceive working in an accident and emergency unit or how they feel about their colleagues, their work, their training and so on. Much has been written about the personal construct approach and the use of the repertory grid technique in research, and the reader is referred to that for further information. It has been used successfully in a number of nursing projects.

SUGGESTED FURTHER READING

Fransella, F. (ed.) (2005) *The Essential Practitioner's Handbook of Personal Construct Psychology.* Chichester: Wiley, pp. 67–76.

Fransella, F., Bell, R. & Bannister, D (2003) *A Manual for Repertory Grid Technique* (2nd edn). Chichester: Wiley.

Jankowicz, A. D. (2003) *The Easy Guide to Repertory Grids.* Chichester: Wiley, pp. 8–31.

Ralley, C., Allott, R., Hare, D.J., Wittkowski, A. (2009) The use of the repertory grid technique to examine staff beliefs about clients with dual diagnosis. *Clinical Psychology & Psychotherapy* 16(2): 148–58.

EXERCISE 6.7

Aim of the exercise: To explore some basic principles of the repertory grid technique.

Planning stage: You can do this exercise on your own or in the company of a small group of colleagues, friends or students. Allow yourself plenty of time to complete the exercise and make notes of what you do, as you go. If you work with friends or colleagues, decide whether you will all carry out similar tasks or whether you will divide up the work between you.

What to do: Consider the following list of types of people and put a name next to each:

1. A good friend

2. Your mother

3. Your father

4. A favourite teacher

5. Someone you do not like

6. Yourself.

This list is a list of 'elements' for you to consider.

Now think about those elements in threes, as listed below. Consider each of the three elements and identify the ways in which *two* of the people are similar and *different* from the third. In each case, write down the *similarity* and the *difference* in the space provided. This will produce a list of bipolar constructs and will offer you some ideas about how you, as an individual, tend to view people. It is notable that another person's list of constructs will be different from yours.

Three elements for comparison	Similarity (the emerging set of bipolar constructs)	Difference
1, 2, 3		
4, 5, 6		
2, 3, 4		
1, 2, 6		
2, 5, 3		
3, 4, 6		

Now consider the range of personal constructs that have been elicited through this exercise. Are you surprised by the constructs or are they representative of the sorts of qualities that you imagined that you attributed to other people? Compare your findings with those of a colleague and identify the ways in which they are similar and different.

It is worth noting that there are numerous and sophisticated ways of processing the information obtained in this sort of way. For further details of the ways in which this is done, see the references to repertory grid techniques offered in the 'Suggested further reading' section, above.

Critical incident technique

By the end of this section you will have discovered:

■ How to consider using the critical incident technique.

Critical incident technique

Critical incident technique, in its simplest form, offers the opportunity to discover how people say they have reacted in certain situations. For example, it may be useful to find out how nursing assistants felt about how they acted in the event of a patient having a cardiac arrest. It may also be used to discover how different *groups* of people say they reacted in particular situations. For example, it may be interesting to find out how doctors, senior nurses *and* nursing assistants consider how they acted in the event of a patient having a cardiac arrest.

The critical incident technique is used to help people to reflect on past events and to note how they report their reactions to such events. Thus, a group of student nurses may be asked to describe how they dealt with their first experience of a patient having an epileptic fit.

Different methods of data collection may be used to gather examples of incidents for review and for identifying people's perceptions of those incidents. For example, the researcher may use interviews, questionnaires, records and self-report measures.

The analysis of the data obtained involves the classification of people's responses to incidents into particular categories. For example, senior nurses may be asked to think of a time when they were functioning particularly well in their role as teacher. The words and phrases that they use to describe their performance are then filtered into a variety of categories, for example 'effective communication', 'skilled behaviour', 'enjoyment' and so on. These categories can then be used to present the data in a written format and they may allow the researcher to offer answers to the research question.

SUGGESTED FURTHER READING

Kemppainen, J. K. (2001) The critical incident technique and nursing care quality research. *Journal of Advanced Nursing* 32(5): 1264–71.

Keatinge, D. (2002) Versatility and flexibility: Attributes of the critical incident technique in nursing research. *Nursing & Health Sciences* 4(1–2): 33–9.

Narayanasamy, A., Clissett, P., Parumal, L., Thompson, D., Annasamy, S. & Edge, R. (2004) Responses to the spiritual needs of older people. *Journal of Advanced Nursing* 48(1): 6–16.

Schluter, J., Seaton, P. & Chaboyer, W. (2008) Critical incident technique: A user's guide for nursing researchers. *Journal of Advanced Nursing* 61(1): 107–14.

Flanagan, J. C. (1954) The critical incident technique. *Psychological Bulletin* 51(4): 327–58 (a classic paper describing the use of this technique).

EXERCISE 6.8

Aim of the exercise: To explore one aspect of the critical incident technique.

What to do: Consider one of the following incidents from your past:

■ Observing patient having an epileptic fit;

■ The fire alarm sounding when you were at work;

■ Giving a patient an injection;

■ Being present at a road traffic accident.

Now write down what happened and write down *what you did*. Now consider the following questions:

■ Do you consider that your action was appropriate?

■ If not, why not?

■ How did you feel about what happened?

■ In what ways could your performance have been improved?

■ What did you learn from the incident?

■ What would you do differently next time?

Now look through your responses and see whether certain trends occur and see whether those trends can be placed under certain broad headings.

Multiple sorting technique

By the end of this section you will have discovered:

■ Whether the multiple sort technique may be suitable for your project.

The multiple sort method combines two other sorts of data collection methods: the 'Q' sort (Stephenson 1953) and the repertory grid approach, described above. The exercise that follows explains the basic principles of the method.

EXERCISE 6.9

Aim of the exercise: To explore the use of the multiple sort technique.

What to do: Write the following phrases onto separate cards:

PSYCHIATRIC NURSING   CARDIAC NURSING
GERIATRIC NURSING   MIDWIFERY
PAEDIATRIC NURSING   HEALTH VISITING
ORTHOPAEDIC NURSING   DISTRICT NURSING
OPHTHALMIC NURSING   MACMILLAN NURSING
ONCOLOGY NURSING   COMMUNITY PSYCHIATRIC NURSING

UROLOGICAL NURSING	SCHOOL NURSING
MENTAL HANDICAP NURSING	OCCUPATIONAL HEALTH NURSING
MEDICAL NURSING	INDUSTRIAL NURSING
SURGICAL NURSING	

Now ask your colleague to look through the cards and sort them into piles. The piles may represent any sort of differentiation at all. Your colleague is free to determine how she divides them up. Then ask your colleague to *Label* the piles that she has produced.

Make a note of the labels of the piles and the cards within each pile. Now have a go at sorting the cards yourself. See whether you produce a different set of piles and, perhaps, a different number of piles.

In doing this exercise you have been using the multiple sort technique: a technique that allows you to explore another person's viewpoint, style of differentiating between things and so forth. Discuss the piles and their labels with your colleague and discuss ways that the method could be used in a research project.

The multiple sorting technique may be used for structuring an interview and collecting qualitative information. It has the distinct advantage of providing a structured interview format and statistical analysis procedure while at the same time it allows the informant to dictate what the important issues and considerations are. In so doing, it allows the researcher to gather rich details about the informant's views of the world, which may be analysed both qualitatively and quantitatively.

The multiple sorting technique is a method which can be used to explore the important constructs which people use to structure and describe their experiences, by examining how they assign elements to conceptual categories. In effect, the multiple sorting technique allows the researcher to study individual perceptions of a specific research topic in a highly structured and organized manner. The 'Suggested further reading' section that follows provides some examples of how the sorting technique has been adapted in different contexts.

SUGGESTED FURTHER READING

Coxon, A. P. M (1999) *Sorting Data: Collection and Analysis.* London: Sage Publication (an essential text for those intending to use MST).

Doney, R. M. & Packer, T. L. (2008) Measuring changes in activity participation of older Australians: Validation of the Activity Card Sort-Australia. *Australian Journal of Ageing* 27(1): 33–7.

Neufeld, A., Harrison, M. J., Rempel, G. R., Larocque, S., Dublin, S., Stewart, M. & Hughes, K. (2004) Practical issues in using a card sort in a study of non-support and family care-giving. *Qualitative Health Research* 14: 1418–28.

Spencer, D. (2009) *Card Sorting: Designing Usable Categories.* Brooklyn, NY: Rosenfeld Media (an excellent introduction with lots of practical advice and spreadsheet downloads).

Use of existing scales, inventories, tests and assessment tools

By the end of this section you will have discovered:

- How to find existing scales, inventories, tests and assessment tools;
- Whether such scales, inventories, tests or assessment tools would be useful in your research project.

================ **EXERCISE 6.10** ================

Aim of the exercise: To explore the use of pre-existing scales, inventories and assessment tools.

What to do: Go to the library and locate one or more of the following sources of established scales, inventories, tests or assessment tools:

Bowling, A. (2001) *Measuring Disease. A Review of Disease Specific Quality of Life Measurement Scales* (2nd edn). Buckingham: Open University Press/McGraw-Hill.

Bowling, A. (2004) *Measuring Health: A Review of Quality of Life Measurement Scales* (3rd edn). Milton Keynes: Open University Press.

Olin, J. T. & Keatinge, C. (1998) *Rapid Psychological Assessment*. New York: Wiley.

Tansella, M. & Thornicroft, G. (eds) (2001) *Mental Health Outcome Measures* (2nd edn). London: Gaskell.

Miller, D. C. (2002) *Handbook of Research Design and Social Measurement* (6th edn). Newbury Park: Sage.

McDowell, I. & Newell, C. (1996) *Measuring Health. A Guide to Rating Scales and Questionnaires* (2nd edn). New York: Oxford University Press.

Robinson, J. P., Shaver, P. R. & Wrightman, L.S. (eds) (1991) *Measures of Personality and Social Psychological Attitudes*. San Diego, California: Academic Press.

Scan through two of the instruments that you have found discussed in the literature and answer the following questions:

- How was the instrument developed?

- How was it tested?

- Does the instrument relate specifically to nursing? If not, could it be used in a nursing context?

- Does the instrument relate to a particular culture or does it claim to be applicable across a wide range of different cultures?

- Is it suitable for your particular needs? If not, why not?

- If you were to use it, would you need permission to use it?

- Would you have to pay to use it?

- Could the instrument be 'adapted' for your particular needs?

- Can the instrument be administered by anyone or does the administration need to be supervised by a registered practitioner such as a psychologist?

- Could you analyse the data obtained?

If you find that you *do* want to use a particular instrument, discuss its use with a lecturer first. You may be surprised at how many instruments have already been defined. In addition, you may be able to adapt an existing instrument to suit your particular needs. If a suitable instrument does exist, you may be advised to use it, rather than spend considerable time devising your own. Exploring the types of instruments available will give you some ideas on how established scales and measures look to respondents and what types of scoring systems have been used. If these look friendly and easy to use they are more likely to produce a better response rate. If they look long and complicated then people are less likely to take the time to complete them.

Delphi Method

The Delphi Method is used to quantify the judgements of experts, to assess priorities, or to produce long-range forecasts. Linstone and Turoff

(1975 http://is.njit.edu/pubs/delphibook/) suggest, among other things, that the Delphi Method is useful as a means of:

- Gathering current and historical data not accurately known or available;

- Examining the significance of historical events;

- Evaluating possible budget options;

- Exploring planning options;

- Planning curriculum developments;

- Looking at the pros and cons of policy options.

The Delphi Method, in essence, involves the asking of a group of experts in a particular field to offer information about a particular topic. Out of the material that is generated, a questionnaire is developed, which is then sent out to that same panel of experts. This cyclical process is continued until the researcher feels confident that she is obtaining a reasonably comprehensive view of the field. The aim is to produce an outcome that is acceptable to the panel of experts.

SUGGESTED FURTHER READING

Hardy, D. J., O'Brien, A. P., Gaskin, C. J., O'Brien, A. J., Morrison-Ngatai, E., Skews, G., Ryan, T. & McNulty, N. (2004) Practical application of the Delphi Technique in a bicultural mental health nursing study in New Zealand. *Journal of Advanced Nursing* 46(1): 95–109.

Keeney, S., Hasson, F. & McKenna, H. (2006) Consulting the oracle: Ten lessons from using the Delphi technique in nursing research. *Journal of Advanced Nursing* 53(2): 205–12.

Powell, C. (2003) The Delphi technique: Myths and realities. *Journal of Advanced Nursing* 41(4): 376–82.

Vernon, W. (2009) The Delphi technique: A review. *International Journal of Therapy and Rehabilitation* 16(2): 69–76.

The above are just some of the methods that you might like to explore. There are lots more to learn about if you have the time and energy to do so. Our intention here was to offer up examples of some commonly used and some not so commonly used methods in studies of nurses and nursing. Perhaps the overriding principle in selecting a method is that it should be the one that most clearly offers you the data that can answer your research question or help to solve your research problem.

CONCLUSION

In this chapter we have considered four main types of data collection methods and some other less frequently used methods. If you can become familiar with the essential elements of the four main types you will be better able to examine, critically, the research literature. The other methods have not been used as frequently in nursing research but all offer interesting and valuable methods of collecting data.

It is wise to become familiar with a wide range of such methods and to note how other researchers, before you, have chosen their methods. In this way you will gradually become more critical of other people's work: a vital aspect of the research process.

Choosing a Data Collection Method

7

AIMS OF THIS CHAPTER

- To clarify which method of data collection you aim to use in your project;

- To clarify how your data is going to be analysed after collection.

Introduction

In the previous chapter we discussed in some depth the different data collection methods available for you to choose. The time has come to make a decision about which you think will be the most suitable to collect the data to answer your research question and that best fits with your research design. If you feel that you do not have sufficient information about certain of the methods to be able to make a decision, refer to other texts and journal articles that will help you to understand these methods and assess their suitability.

One word of caution. It is vital that you are clear about how you will *process* your data when you have collected it. Most researchers will be able to tell you horror stories of people who have collected masses of data only to be able to sit back and wonder what to do with it. In planning your method of data collection, you must select your method of analysis at the same time.

Identifying a range of available data collection methods

By the end of this section you will have discovered:

- A range of data collection methods available to you.

======================= **EXERCISE 7.1** =======================

Aim of the exercise: To allow you to consider the range of possible data collection methods that will help you to answer your research question.

What to do: Look through the list of data collection methods in Figure 7.1. Beside each one, use the following code and mark the second column accordingly:

1. Suited to my project;

2. Possibly suited to my project;

3. Unsuited to my project;

4. I do not have enough information about this method to make a decision.

For example, if you feel that the interview method is a suitable one for your project, you put a 1 in the second column. If you feel that the questionnaire method is unsuited to your project, you put a 3 in the second column. If you feel that you do not know enough about the Q sort technique, put a 4 in column 2 and so on.

DATA COLLECTION METHOD	SUITABILITY FOR MY STUDY
Questionnaire	
Interview	
Experiments	
Observation	
Use of existing records	
Repertory grid technique	
Critical incident technique	
Multiple sorting technique	
Use of existing scales (attitude scales, personality inventories, assessment scales etc...)	
Delphi technique	
Other methods you have identified	

Figure 7.1 Matching data collection methods to your study

Evaluation: On what basis did you make your decisions? Do you have enough information to choose your method, at this stage, or do you need to do further studying? Does the data collection method you might choose suit the type of research you are doing, for example, quantitative or qualitative? What does this exercise tell you about some of the problems of collecting data? (The marks you awarded in the above column are data.) What could you do to analyse this data?

Choosing your data collection method

By the end of this section you will have discovered:

■ How to choose a data collection method for your project.

EXERCISE 7.2

Aim of the exercise: To enable you to make a choice about the method you will use to collect your research data.

What to do: Note the methods that you have selected out from the last exercise as being suitable for your project. Now ask yourself the following questions about each method in order to be clearer about the choice you are going to make:

1. Do I know enough about the method?
   (a) If Y, proceed to next item.
   (b) If N, go to the library, read more about the method, and discuss it with your supervisor or someone who has had experience in this field OR proceed to next chapter.

2. Can I justify using this method rather than another?
   (a) If Y, proceed to next item.
   (b) If N, is this through lack of knowledge about other methods? If Y, read up on other methods. If N, proceed to next question in this chain. Is it because I could use a variety of methods? If Y, proceed to next item and keep a range of options open.

3. Have I got the skills to carry out the method?
   (a) If Y, proceed to next item.
   (b) If N, find out what the skills are from the library or from a supervisor.

4. Is special equipment required to use this method?

(a) If Y, have I access to it? If N, can I get access? If N, abandon this method.

(b) If N, proceed to next item.

5. Does the method take considerable time to use?

   (a) If Y, have I got the time within my time schedule? If Y, proceed to next item. If N, abandon method.

   (b) If N, proceed to next item.

6. Does the method require a large sample? Before answering this question, read around the question of sampling and discuss it with your supervisor.

   (a) If Y, Have I got access to the number required? If Y, proceed to next item. If N, abandon method.

   (b) If N, proceed to next item.

7. Do I know someone who has used this method and can give me support?

   (a) If Y, proceed with your project.

   (b) If N, Can I find someone? If Y, proceed with your project. If N, proceed with caution!

Evaluation: These are some of the questions that must be asked before you proceed with your project. Go to a supervisor and ask them to quiz you on your chosen method. Ask a colleague to act as 'devil's advocate' and ask you particularly awkward questions about the method.

   The final and *most important* question must be: Is this method the most appropriate one for answering your research question? It may be tempting to ignore or rush through this process of clear decision-making but it is folly to do so. As you work through the process as described above it will help you to choose a method of data collection that is grounded in earlier studies and well suited to your particular project. You will also be able to provide a sound rationale for this approach in your write up.

Choosing your method of data analysis

By the end of this section you will have discovered:

■ The appropriate data analysis method for your research project.

As we noted earlier, it is vital that you consider how you will analyse your data as you collect it. This decision must be made alongside the decision about which data collection method you are going to use and not after that decision.

====== **EXERCISE 7.3** ======

Aim of the exercise: To help you to decide whether the most appropriate method of analysis for your data is qualitative or quantitative or a mixture of both.

What to do:

Consider the following questions:

At the end of your data collection are you going to have data

■ which is easily converted into numbers? (e.g. A person may be asked to state whether they agree or disagree with a set of attitude statements in which the range of responses is: strongly disagree, disagree, uncertain, agree and strongly agree. These response labels can be given numerical values as follows: SD=1, D=2, UC=3, A=4, SA=5. These numbers can then be totalled and statistic procedures used to identify trends in the data.)

OR

■ in the form of text or other 'blocks' of words (e.g. a series of interview transcripts or a series of passages taken from books, documents, records, etc.)?

OR

■ which includes both numbers and text? If so, read and work through both of the sections below.

If your project will lead you to numbers, consider the following questions:

■ Are you clear about how you will collect and store your data? Remember ethics committees have specific storage requirements.

■ Do you have the necessary skills to perform the statistical analysis required in processing the data?

■ If statistical tests are required, do you know which ones they are and can you use them?

■ Where can you obtain further statistical advice?

■ Do you know how to interpret statistical data?

■ Do you know the limitations of using figures as data?

■ How will you present your figures when you write up your report?

■ Are there short courses in numerical analysis that you could attend?

Now read the relevant chapters in: Bell, J. (2005) *Doing Your Research Project: A Guide For First-Time Researchers in Education and Social Science* (4th edn). Milton Keynes: Oxford University Press.

If your project will lead you to the production of text, consider the following questions:

■ Are you clear about how you will collect and store your data?

■ Do you have the necessary skills to analyse and categorize the data?

■ Where can you obtain further advice on handling textual data?

■ What psychological, sociological or political theories will guide your analysis?

■ Do you know how to interpret any findings?

■ Do you know the limitations of using raw text as data?

■ How will you present your data when your write up your report?

■ Are there short courses or qualitative analysis tools you could use?

Now read chapters 7–11 in: Davies, M. B. (2007) *Doing a Successful Research Project: Using Qualitative or Quantitative Methods.* Basingstoke: Palgrave Macmillan.

Pilot studies

Now that you have considered a variety of methods of collecting data, you may want to 'try out' one or more methods. This will usually lead you to doing a pilot study.

A pilot study is a very small-scale version of the research project which allows you to test out your data collection method and allows you to preview the sort of data that the method will collect for you. It should point up deficiencies in your planning and development of the data collection method and will enable you to smooth out such deficiencies. Alternatively, it may show you that the method you have chosen is not suitable for your project. In this case you may have to go back to the drawing board and consider other methods. Then, of course, you will have to conduct another pilot study. The details of the pilot study should always be written into your final research report and indicate how this 'dummy run' led to changes in the procedures used eventually. Not all research studies require a pilot study but time spent at this stage can pay great dividends later on. Some of the questions that a pilot study will allow you to consider are:

- Can the respondents understand what is being asked of them?

- Does the data collection method collect the sort of data I want?

- Have I got time to use this method?

- Are there unexpected ethical problems associated with this method? Note that you will need ethical approval to conduct a pilot study too.

- Do I know how to analyse the data that this method generates?

- What revisions are required to modify my plan?

CONCLUSION

The choice of method for collecting the sort of information you need is not an easy one and embraces a whole range of issues that we have covered across several chapters in this book. In order to do a project however you have to make some choices and frequently that means leaving behind approaches and ideas that have appealed to you. Whatever the nature of your project, there will always be boundaries and resource issues as you attempt to complete a study in a real world setting. Making informed choices about the design, data collection and analysis methods will help to ensure that your project is of sound quality within these parameters. Every project is limited in some important ways.

Methods of Analysing Data

8

AIMS OF THIS CHAPTER

- Examine methods of analysing data quantitatively;

- Examine methods of analysing data qualitatively;

- Explore combinations of the two approaches;

- Aid the selection of an appropriate method of data analysis for your project.

Introduction

In the previous chapters, we considered the various methods of collecting data that are available to the researcher. We noted also, that very often the data collection method is intimately tied to the method of analysis – hence we asked you to identify whether your data collection method was more likely to lend itself to quantitative, qualitative or a mixture of both data analysis methods. This raises the very important issue that has been alluded to before: methods of analysis must always be considered alongside methods of data collection.

In this chapter we consider two broad approaches to data analysis:

- quantitative and

- qualitative.

Before you work through this chapter, it may be helpful to re-read the sections on the differences between quantitative and qualitative approaches to research, outlined in chapter 4. You will recall that an important difference, in terms of outcome, was that *quantitative* research tends to generate data in the form of numbers. *Qualitative* research tends to generate data that is made up of blocks of text that are interpreted in various ways. The purpose of the analysis, in both cases, however, is to identify patterns or trends emerging from the data. In addition, the researcher must carry out various checks to ensure that these patterns or trends are both *reliable* and *valid* findings (see chapter 5). In this chapter, the two types of data analysis, quantitative and qualitative are discussed separately. In the conclusion to this chapter, we explore, briefly, the notion of combining the two approaches.

Quantitative analysis

SUGGESTED READING

This should include several of the following:

Bell, J. (2005) *Doing Your Research Project: A Guide for First-Time Researchers in Education and Social Science* (4th edn). Milton Keynes : Open University Press, pp. 201–30.

Mantzoukas, S. (2009) The research evidence published in high impact nursing journals between 2000–2006: A quantitative content analysis. *International Journal of Nursing Studies* 46(4): 479–89.

Polit, D. & Beck, C. (2010) *Essentials of Nursing Research: Appraising Evidence for Nursing Practice*. Philadelphia: Lippincott Williams & Wilkins, pp. 392–439.

Reeve, J., James, F. & McNeill, R. (2009) Providing psychosocial and physical rehabilitation advice for patients with burns. *Journal of Advanced Nursing* 65(5): 1039–43.

Robson, C. (2002) *Real World Research: A Resource for Social Scientists and Practitioner-Researchers* (2nd edn). Oxford: Wiley-Blackwell, pp. 391–455.

Salkind, N. (2007) *Statistics for People who (think they) Hate Statistics* (2nd edn). London: Sage (There is no particular section of this book; rather peruse the contents and index to target your reading).

Taylor, J., Lauder, W., Moy, M. & Collett, J. (2009) Practitioner assessments of "good enough" preventing: Factorial survey. *Journal of Clinical Nursing* 18(8): 1180–9.

Types of quantitative analysis

By the end of this section you will have discovered:

- Some common terms used in quantitative analysis;
- Some of the common tests used in quantitative analysis;
- Whether any of these methods are useful to you in analysing your data.

═══════════════════ **EXERCISE 8.1** ═══════════════════

Aim of the exercise: To explore common terms used in quantitative analysis.

What to do: Go to the library and select a range of books on research methods. Then consider the terms below and write short notes on what they mean. The books recommended above will help you to make a start on this task.

- Statistics: descriptive and inferential
- Nominal scales
- Ordinal scales
- Interval scales
- Ratio scales
- Variable
- Discrete and continuous variable
- Mean
- Mode
- Standard deviation
- Normal distribution
- Parametric and non-parametric tests
- Median
- Cumulative frequency.

Note down other words that are unfamiliar to you and describe their meanings. If you are working in a group discuss your findings with others.

Now find examples from the literature of the following ways of presenting numerical data:

- Graph
- Pie charts
- Tables
- Histograms
- Bar charts
- Percentage component bar chart
- Statistical significance
- Probability
- *t*-test
- Chi-square test
- Pearson correlation coefficient.

Discuss your findings and your progress with your colleagues and a lecturer. What sort of data do you think your research project will generate? Consider to what degree quantitative methods of analysis will be appropriate for your project. If not, consider the extent to which you will need to understand this approach to analysis to be able to critically evaluate research reports you read. Reflect on some of the advantages and disadvantages of the quantitative approach and link your discussion of these issues with the earlier chapter in this book which compares and contrasts the two approaches to research.

Quantitative analysis

Quantitative analysis is nearly always analysis of figures. Usually the easiest way of working with lots of figures is by putting them into 'rows and columns'. For this reason, a computer is often the best way of working with numerical data. At least two possibilities open up here. First, numerical data can be stored and, to some extent, manipulated with a spreadsheet program. A spreadsheet program allows you to enter numbers into series of rows and columns and then to perform simple and complex calculations on those rows and columns – Some spreadsheet programs come with a data analysis module that allows for some statistical computations. The findings from those calculations can be converted into a variety of tables and charts or even transferred into a word processing program for further work.

The alternative to working with a spreadsheet is to put your numerical data into a statistical analysis program. This works in a similar way to a spreadsheet application but it also allows for the use of far more complex statistical calculations such as the statistical package for the social sciences (SPSS) (more on this towards the end of the chapter). Again, all of these programs allow you to produce charts and tables from your findings. An important point is that you should always know *why* you are using a particular statistical test before you ask the program to run it. Computer programs will run statistical tests on any lists of figures but the results of indiscriminate computing can lead to findings that are nonsensical.

The principles of quantitative analysis can be simplified as follows:

1st stage: Findings are grouped together in rows and columns. This is sometimes referred to as the presentation of 'raw' data.

2nd stage: The researcher looks for consistent trends and patterns in the data and sees how the findings are distributed throughout the sample. Descriptive statistics can be used here in the form of frequency counts, means, modes and standard deviations.

3rd stage: The researcher looks for *particular* trends, patterns and relationships between variables. For example, he or she may look at differences between sexes or age groups. The researcher may use a range of statistical tests to verify his or her findings.

4th stage: The researcher presents the findings in a series of charts or tables.

5th stage: The researcher offers *interpretations* or *explanations* of the findings and writes the final research report to communicate the findings which address the research questions.

These are only *general* guidelines. You need to read more widely on all the possible stages that a quantitative researcher may use in analysing the data.

Example

The following short questionnaire is given to 20 people. Each respondent fills in his or her questionnaire and each question on the questionnaire has five possible answers. The first possible answer (strongly agree) is assigned a '1', the second possible answer (agree) is assigned a '2', the third possible answer (uncertain) is assigned a '3' and so on. The example, below, shows how one respondent filled in the questionnaire.

1. Primary nursing is a useful way of organizing nursing work.

Strongly Agree	Agree	Uncertain	Disagree	Strongly Disagree	LEAVE BLANK
1 ✓	2	3	4	5	

2. All nurses should use a nursing model to plan their nursing care.

Strongly Agree	Agree	Uncertain	Disagree	Strongly Disagree	LEAVE BLANK
1 ✓	2	3	4	5	

3. Student nurses generally receive excellent training in the use of nursing models.

Strongly Agree	Agree	Uncertain	Disagree	Strongly Disagree	LEAVE BLANK
1	2 ✓	3	4	5	

4. Nursing models are unnecessarily complicated.

Strongly Agree	Agree	Uncertain	Disagree	Strongly Disagree	LEAVE BLANK
1 ✓	2	3	4	5	

5. Primary nursing is not an appropriate approach to nursing in the community.

Strongly Agree	Agree	Uncertain	Disagree	Strongly Disagree	LEAVE BLANK
1	2	3	4 ✓	5	

After all the questionnaires have been filled in, the researcher 'scores' them by inserting the number of the ticked box in the 'leave blank' box. This facility is particularly useful if large numbers of questionnaires are being handled.

Once all the questionnaire items have been scored in this way, the researcher transfers all the scores to the main score sheet. This makes use of the 'rows and columns' arrangement referred to above. The numbered grid allows all of the answers to each question in all of the questionnaires to be grouped together in a single sheet. Alternatively, these numbers could be typed into a spreadsheet or statistics program on a computer (Table 8.1). Any 'missing' score (where the respondent has missed answering a particular item) is allocated the number 9 to distinguish it from any 'actual' answers.

After this, the researcher can determine, either by hand or through the use of a computer, a 'frequency count'. This means that he or she works out how many '5's there were as a response to question 1 (and, therefore, how many people answered 'strongly disagree' to it), how many '4's and so on. From this type of frequency count, if he had a large

Table 8.1 Example of a spreadsheet showing responses to five questions involving 20 responses

Respondent Number	Quest 1	Quest 2	Quest 3	Quest 4	Quest 5
R1	1	1	2	1	4
R2	2	1	4	3	3
R3	2	2	4	3	3
R4	1	2	5	4	3
R5	3	2	5	2	3
R6	1	2	5	1	1
R7	3	3	5	3	9
R8	1	2	4	1	2
R9	2	4	2	1	2
R10	1	1	5	1	1
R11	2	3	3	3	4
R12	1	5	5	1	5
R13	1	3	9	1	5
R14	1	3	5	3	2
R15	4	3	4	3	3
R16	4	2	4	2	4
R17	2	4	5	4	1
R18	3	9	9	3	4
R19	1	2	3	1	1
R20	2	1	4	1	1

number of responses, he could work out the *percentage* of respondents' responses to all of the questionnaire items. After this, he could illustrate those percentages in a *bar chart*. Figure 8.1 shows a frequency count for question 1, from the above grid.

It is easy to see how all the '5's, all the '4's, '3's, '2's and '1's in each column could be calculated and how '9's would have to be discounted. It may also be easy to see how items of data soon mount up. This was a very short questionnaire given to a small number of respondents and yet it yielded 100 separate items of data. Larger questionnaires and larger samples of respondents are nearly always more easily handled with a computer program.

These data could also be analysed in other ways. Let us assume for a moment that the list of questions made up a scale to measure attitudes to nursing models and presented this to respondents so that high scores indicated a positive attitude and low scores indicated a negative attitude.

Question 1: Primary nursing is a useful way of organizing nursing work.	Numbers of responses
Strongly agree (1's)	9
Agree (2's)	6
Uncertain (3's)	3
Disagree (4's)	2
Strongly disagree (5's)	0
Total number of responses	20

Figure 8.1 Example of a frequency count table showing responses to question 1 in exercise example

In this scenario we would be able to add the scores on each question-naire item for each respondent (row scores) and the total score and then the average score for each item in the questionnaire (columns). This would provide us with a much richer picture of the data and lead us to ask more questions.

EXERCISE 8.2

Aim of the exercise: To explore some simple statistical calculations.

What to do: Consider the following table:

Monthly discharge rate from an acute admission psychiatric ward over a two-year period.

Months of the year

	J	F	M	A	M	J	J	A	S	O	N	D
Year 1	27	24	30	30	21	24	29	28	20	25	24	22
Year 2	29	30	26	24	20	29	30	24	22	23	23	20

Now calculate the following:

■ The mean discharge rate over the two-year period.

■ The mean discharge rate for year one and for year two.

■ The mean discharge rate for each month of the year, over the two-year period.

Now draw a bar chart that illustrates the mean discharge rate for each month of the year, over the two-year period.

Now calculate the following:

- The frequency of each of the values, Convert these into a pie chart.

- Now calculate:

- The median for this set of values;

- The cumulative frequency for this set of values.

If you experience any problems with these calculations, refer to:

Bell, J. (2005) *Doing Your Research Project: A Guide For First-Time Researchers in Education and Social Science* (4th edn). Milton Keynes: Oxford University Press, pp. 201–30.

or

Polit, D. & Beck, C. (2010) *Essentials of Nursing Research: Appraising Evidence for Nursing Practice*. Philadelphia: Lippincott Williams & Wilkins, pp. 392–439.

EXERCISE 8.3

Aim of the exercise: To explore problems associated with the use of statistical arguments.

What to do: Read the following proposition and the rationale that accompanies it. The rationale offers an explanation of a statistical table and the proposition is based on how a statistician can interpret a set of statistics. Read the passage through and then decide for yourself if the proposition is a valid one. If you come to the conclusion that it is, think again!

This is an exercise in the art of reading statistics. The discussion focuses on one proposition and is divided into two parts. The first offers a statistical argument in support of the proposition. The second offers a critique of that statistical argument. The critique is developed by noting any assumptions, inconsistencies or fallacies in the statistical argument and building the discussion around them.

The art of reading statistics is to place them in an appropriate context and then to interpret them by reference to that background. This requires considerable knowledge of the relevant subject areas, so read the discussions critically and carefully!

The proposition: Marriage is fatal for the man

The Supporting Argument It is no longer socially unacceptable for a couple to enter into an unhallowed and extra-legal partnership in which they live together as man and wife. This change in attitude developed from the appreciation by a substantial proportion of adults of the real consequences of marriage. It is, quite simply, that marriage is fatal for the man. The table below demonstrates this fact conclusively.

Women outnumber men. However, they do not do so over all age groups. In the younger age group men outnumber women. As men grow older this situation is reversed by their death rate increasing more rapidly than the death rate for women. The change occurs when men and women are in the fifth decade of their lives. Its effect is that a 3 per cent surplus of men in the younger age group is converted to a 23 per cent surplus of women in the older age groups.

A single factor produces the change. A common experience of the factor kills men more quickly than women. That factor is marriage. Is it sufficiently widespread to produce the change? And, by the time the change occurs men have experienced marriage for a sufficient length of time for it to produce the change. The extent of the change is accounted for by the virulence of marriage.

Now evaluate the above argument, either as individuals working alone or with colleagues or friends in a group setting. Can you spot any problems in the above set of arguments? Do not give up too quickly. The development of critical skills is an important one. If you cannot puzzle out the problems, read the paragraphs below. If you do identify problems, read the paragraphs to confirm your own arguments or to develop other perspectives on the problem.

Table 8.2 Population of England and Wales, mid-1971 ('000s)

Age	Male	Female	Total
0–4	2 009	1 911	3 920
5–14	3 980	3 776	7 756
15–19	1 715	1 640	3 355
20–29	3 526	3 469	6 995
30–44	4 340	4 258	8 598
45–74	7 437	8 506	15 943
75 and over	713	1 534	2 247
Totals	23 720	25 094	48 814

Source: *The Registrar General's Statistical Review of England and Wales, 1971*, part 2, 1973, Table A6: 10–11. Reproduced under the Open Government Licence v1.0.

A critique of the supporting argument

The statistical argument implies that the table shows what happened over time. But the table shows the situation at a single point in time, namely, mid-1971. It therefore does not show that 'as men grow older … a 3 per cent surplus of men in the younger age groups is converted into a 23 per cent surplus of women in the older age groups'. The only statistics which can show whether such a conversion occurs are those which compare the same group of men and women over all age groups. They are obtained by following the group throughout its life.

As an illustration of what such statistics would show, consider the '75 and over' age group. It contains the largest surplus of women. Notice that a man aged 75 years in 1971 would have been 20 years old in 1916, that is, about the middle of the First World War. Clearly, the surplus of women is explained, in part at least, by the ravages on the battlefields of that war.

Now consider the second oldest age group. It is the only other age group in which women outnumber men. Notice that a man aged 50 years in 1971 would have been 20 years old in 1942: this is near the middle of the Second World War. Once again, the surplus of women is explained, in part at least, by battlefield deaths.

In both age groups the differences are further reduced by the residual effects of the two wars. These effects include the premature deaths of men who survived the wars as battlefield casualties and as prisoners of war. They also include the premature deaths of men who were not conscripted because of ill health.

The statistical argument states that 'a common experience … kills men more quickly than women'. This implies that a causal relationship exists when two factors are each experienced by a large proportion of the individuals in a group. In other words, it implies that a strong statistical relationship denotes a causal relationship. In fact, a strong statistical relationship does nothing of the kind. All any statistical relationship can ever do is show the observed strength of a causal relationship established by theory. The reason is quite simple. Statistical relationships are easy to manufacture.

As an example, suppose that in a group of 10 women, 8 are married and 8 wear jeans. At least 6, that is, at least 75 per cent of the married women wear jeans. Consequently, there is a strong statistical relationship between being married and wearing jeans. As this is a fabricated relationship, it is quite meaningless, despite its apparent strength. If this were not so, the relationship would show that only married women normally wear jeans. In this case the converse would also be true. This is that single women do not normally wear jeans. We know that neither is true.

Clearly, the statistical argument supporting the notion that marriage is fatal for men is defective on two major counts. It is also defective on a third count. The data are inappropriate. The comparison should be of married men and women, not all men and women. And, the measure of the effect of marriage should be the length of marriage at death, not the age of the individual.

Individually the deficiencies raise doubts about the validity of the statistical argument. Together they establish that it is totally unsound. The statistical argument therefore does not support the proposition. It does not establish that marriage is fatal for the man, even though this may well be the case.

Qualitative analysis

SUGGESTED READING

This should include the following:

Anthony, S. & Jack, S. (2009) Qualitative case study methodology in nursing research: An integrative review. *Journal of Advanced Nursing* 65(6): 1171–81.

Barredo, RDV & Dudley, T. J. (2008) A descriptive study of losses associated with permanent long-term care placement. *Journal of Geriatric Physical Therapy* 31(3): 87–92.

Crang, M. & Cook, I. (2007) *Doing Ethnographies*. London: Sage..

Flick, U. (2007) *Designing Qualitative Research*. London: Sage, pp. 100–8.

Lyneham, J., Parkinson, C. & Denholm, C. (2008) Intuition in emergency nursing: A phenomenological study. *International Journal of Nursing Practice* 14: 101–8.

McBrien, B. (2008) Evidence-based care: Enhancing the rigour of a qualitative study. *British Journal of Nursing* 17(20): 286–9.

Polit, D. & Beck, C. (2010) *Essentials of Nursing Research: Appraising Evidence for Nursing Practice*. Philadelphia: Lippincott Williams & Wilkins, pp. 441–8.

Watkins, M., Jones, R., Lindsey, L. & Sheaff, R. (2008) The clinical content of NHS trust board meetings: An initial exploration. *Journal of Nursing Management* 16(6): 707–15.

Exploring qualitative analysis

By the end of this section you will have discovered:

- How to identify different frameworks for analysing qualitative data;
- Whether any of these methods are useful to you in analysing your data.

Qualitative analysis

Using qualitative data analysis techniques means that the researcher starts with different *sorts* of data to the quantitative researcher. In the main qualitative data nearly always entails working with *text*. Also, the qualitative researcher often starts with a different set of assumptions about the purpose and nature of the research process. The philosophical positions of the two types of research design may or may not be quite different.

In the end, all researchers using a qualitative design have to make sense of what can be large amounts of text – often in the form of transcripts. Like all researchers this involves searching for patterns and groupings in those data, in an attempt to understand what other people think, feel, experience and how they act in particular settings. The problem for the qualitative researcher is staying 'true' to the informant or participant. While quantitative data analysis is dealing with numbers, the qualitative data analysis is dealing with the difficult area of personal meanings. Qualitative data analysis also involves the use of induction, insight and creativity skills to identify themes or patterns in the data.

Just as there are computer programs to help in quantitative analysis, so there are others (see below) that help the researcher to organize and analyse qualitative data. The following stages represent some of the stages that may be worked through by a qualitative researcher:

Stage 1: The data is gathered into a manageable format – usually a series of transcriptions from taped interviews or extensive field notes.

Stage 2: The data is analysed into smaller chunks, meaning units or categories.

Stage 3: The researcher looks for common themes and patterns.

Stage 4: The researcher checks the validity of his or her analysis both with other researchers, with the informants and with the available literature.

Stage 5: The researcher offers accounts and explanations of *why* the data group together in this way or fit with a particular theoretical framework.

Stage 6: If required, the researcher refines old theories in the light of the findings or develops new theories.

Stage 8: The researcher writes up and communicates the findings.

These are only *general* guidelines. You need to read more widely on all the possible stages that a qualitative researcher may use in analysing his or her data.

Example

Ten semi-structured interviews were conducted with nursing lecturers and extracts from two interviews are illustrated below. The interviews were about assessing teaching in a college of nursing.

Extract one

RESEARCHER: *... and what sorts of methods of assessment do you use, yourself?*

INTERVIEWEE: *I ask the students, I suppose. I ask them at the end of the block of study how they felt about the teaching. I mean, I suppose it's not very scientific ... sometimes I give them a questionnaire to fill in. It's not easy. The books suggest that you should regularly assess your teaching so that you can improve learning but I am not sure that the connection between teaching and learning has been established. Not completely.*

Extract two

RESEARCHER: *... how do you know that the students like your teaching?*

INTERVIEWEE: *They tell me! They tell me that they like the way I do things. That's the most important thing, really – that the students feel OK about what happens. Some of my colleagues use more formal approaches but I'm not sure that they get anything more out of it. One interviews each of the students at the end of the block – a sort of tutorial. I think they tell him what he wants to hear.*

Following the interviews, the researcher read through each of the transcripts and identified a range of categories that appeared to account for *everything* that each interviewee talked about. The complete range of categories was as follows (bear in mind that the two examples, above, are only *small extracts* from *two* of the interviews – in reality a 45-minute interview might lead to at least 10–20 pages of transcript): Student's views of teaching; Lecturer's views of teaching; The 'feel-good' factor; Assessment procedures; Student assessment; Personal preferences; Theories about assessment.

After these categories had been developed, the researcher returned to each of his interview transcripts and divided them up according to those categories. The section below shows how some parts of the extracts above fitted into the category system that had been developed. In 'real life', the process of selecting categories and making sure they are exhaustive of everything that has been discussed in interviews is a laborious and complicated one and one that needs considerable time and concentration. Also, the category system needs to be checked with other colleagues and with the interviewees for face validity. It is important that the category system that you have developed is a valid one and that there is clear evidence that you did not simply 'dream up' the categories. Care has to be taken to ensure that you have not 'massaged' the data to fit with your own beliefs about the topic being studied. The analysis must be rigorous.

Category: The feel-good' factor

'That's the most important thing, really – that the students feel OK about what happens'.

Category: Theories about assessment

'The books suggest that you should regularly assess your teaching so that you can improve learning but I am not sure that the connection between teaching and learning has been established. Not completely'.

Category: Assessment procedures

'I ask the students, I suppose. I ask them at the end of the block of study how they felt about the teaching. I mean, I suppose it's not very scientific…'

'… sometimes I give them a questionnaire to fill in. It's not easy'.

'They tell me! They tell me that they like the way I do things'.

This example is *one* example of a form of *content analysis* of interviews. However, there are many *other* ways of analysing qualitative data. For examples of these read the following articles:

SUGGESTED READING

Barker, C. & Pistrang, N. (2005) Quality criteria under methodological pluralism: Implications for conducting and evaluating research. *American Journal of Community Psychology* 35: 201–12.

Marshall, M., Carter, B., Rose, K. & Brotherton, A. (2009) Living with type 1 diabetes: Perspectives of children and their parents. *Journal of Clinical Nursing* 18(12): 1703–10.

Stein, C. H. & Mankowski, E. S. (2004) Asking, witnessing, interpreting, knowing: Conducting qualitative research in community psychology. *American Journal of Community Psychology* 33: 21–35.

Usher, K., Baker, J. A., Holmes, C. & Stocks, B. (2009) Clinical decision-making for 'as needed' medications in mental health care. *Journal of Advanced Nursing* 65(5): 981–91.

EXERCISE 8.4

Aim of the exercise: To explore qualitative analysis of data.

What to do: Read through the following extract from an interview with a patient. The interview comes from a study of patient's perceptions of the information they have been given about their illness. As you read through, consider what *sorts* of statements the person is making and whether a number of the statements fall into certain groups of themes. For example, does the person refer to certain grades of staff; does she talk about how she feels and so on?

I've been on the ward about six weeks now … no one really tells you very much…I mean, the doctor talked to my husband and my daughter. He didn't talk to me. I get very depressed about it all. Sometimes I don't sleep all that well. Mind you, I don't sleep very well at home, either. The sister's very good. She always answers any questions I have but she doesn't seem to want to talk to me about what's wrong with me.…I think I know though. My daughter always tells me not to worry. I get scared, sometimes. Why won't they tell me?

I go to physiotherapy twice a week. Susan, down there, always says how well I'm doing. I don't think she really knows the whole story. She's more interested in my leg! I like it down there, though … I meet a lot of other people. You can talk to other people because they're in the same boat. I don't get so fed up down there. It's the company, I think. Mind you, my husband tries to talk to me. It's not the same in hospital, though.

The aim of a qualitative analysis of this sort of data is to classify as many statements of units of meaning from the data so that the researcher can make sense of it. The generation of categories of response also allows for comparisons to be made between different sets of data.

Read through the passage above, again, and try to organize phrases from the passage under the following headings that have been generated from the data:

- Types of people discussed
- Feelings expressed
- Activities
- Levels of communication
- Comments about being in hospital
- Comparisons of hospital life with other aspects of life
- Theories about communication in hospital
- Comments about illness.

Example

- Feelings expressed:

  'I get very depressed about it all'
  'I get scared, sometimes'
  'I don't get so fed up down there' (physiotherapy)

This is one stage, in one approach to qualitative analysis.

Now read the following material on qualitative analysis and compare the method you have just explored with other qualitative methods. Also note how the method described here fits into the overall research plan. For example, what could you do after you have discovered categories in the data? How would you write up your analysis?

The reading material is:

Kvale, S. & Brinkman, S. (2009) *Interviews: Learning the Craft of Qualitative Research Interviewing* (2nd edn). London: Sage (a very detailed and rich exploration of the use, type and analysis of qualitative interviews).

Pivik, J., Rode, E. & Ward, C. (2004) A consumer involvement model for health technology assessment in Canada. *Health Policy* 69(2): 253–68.

Using quantitative and qualitative approaches in the same study

Many research projects draw on both quantitative and qualitative ways of collecting and analysing data as a means of developing a richer understanding of the problems and issues being studied – refer back to chapter 4 for an overview of mixed methods. Analysis of the data using both methods is managed in different ways depending on the strategy the researcher has used in the design of the study. In some studies the data collection and thus the data analysis occur concurrently. This approach offers the opportunity to examine the phenomenon being studied from different perspectives. In other studies the quantitative and qualitative data collection and analysis are sequential so that the second phase builds on the first. Whichever type of design is being used the data analysis process of the quantitative and qualitative methods is the same as if they are being used alone. The difference lies in how the findings are then used together to answer the research question/s.

SUGGESTED FURTHER READING

Borbasi, S., Jackson, D. & Langford, R. (2008) *Navigating the Maze of Nursing Research* (2nd edn). Marrackville: Elsevier, pp. 190–4.

Robinson, A., Andrews-Hall, S., Cubit, K., Fassett, M., Venter, L., Menzies, B. & Jongeling, L. (2008) Attracting students to aged care: The impact of a supportive orientation. *Nurse Education Today* 28(3): 354–62.

Zilembo, M. & Monterosso, L. (2008) Nursing students' perceptions of desirable leadership qualities in nurse preceptors: A descriptive survey. *Contemporary Nurse* 27(2): 194–206.

Software for analysis

There are various types of software to help you with your project. If you are a student some software companies offer a student discount if you wish to purchase these. Some examples of programs that perform basic and advanced statistical operations:

http://www.minitab.com/
http://www.spss.com/
http://www.systat.com/
http://www.statsoft.com

Some examples of programs that perform basic analysis and advanced theory building capacities:

http://www.atlasti.com
https://leximancer.thecustomerinsightportal.com/
http://www.provalisresearch.com/

http://www.qualisresearch.com/
http://www.qsrinternational.com/

It is worth remembering that some of the desktop software that is available on most computers these days will have the capacity to undertake quite sophisticated forms of analysis and tests (spreadsheets) or indeed help to search and categorize text files into specific themes (word processing programs).

Learning more about quantitative and qualitative research

These are some routes to learning more about the subject:

- Evening classes at colleges and extra-mural departments of universities;
- Asking for a course of lectures on the topic in the school or college of nursing;
- Using learning packages;
- Working with a research supervisor;
- Reading;
- Open University programmes on the television;
- Lectures and seminar groups;
- Working alongside an experienced researcher;
- Taking part in collecting data for a researcher;
- Volunteering as a respondent in a research project;
- Learning computer programs to analyse data – both qualitative and quantitative.

CONCLUSION

You have now explored two approaches to handling data analysis. From a philosophical point of view, the quantitative and qualitative approaches start from very different assumptions about the nature of research. From a practical point of view, however, it is possible to use and combine both approaches. The choice of data analysis method cannot be made in isolation from the other decisions about research design. In the next chapter, we will bring together everything we have learnt so far about undertaking a research project and discuss how we actually put the research plan into action.

CHAPTER

9

Undertaking the Research Project

AIMS OF THIS CHAPTER

These are to:

- Explore aspects of effective time management

- Explore aspects of supervision

- Aid you to plan and work consistently through your project.

Introduction

All the previous chapters have focused on discrete parts of the research process. Our aim in this chapter is to pull the threads together to enable you to work through the project as a whole.

SUGGESTED READING

Reading a selection from this list will describe different aspects of this chapter.

Bell, J. (2008) *Doing Your Research Project: A Guide for First-time Researchers in Education, Health and Social Science* (4th edn). Berkshire: Open University Press, pp. 28–43.

Gould, D. (2008) Undertaking a research project: Guidance for nursing students. *Nursing Standard* 22(50): 48–54.

Gill, P. & Burnard, P. (2008) The student-supervisor relationship in the PhD/Doctoral process. *British Journal of Nursing* 17(10): 668–71.

Mitchell, T. & Caroll, J. (2008) Academic and research misconduct in the PhD: Issues for students and supervisors. *Nurse Education Today* 28(2): 218–26.

Davies, M. (2007) *Doing a Successful Research Project*. Hampshire: Palgrave McMillan, pp. 36–50.

Robson, C. (2007) *How to Do a Research Project: A Guide for Undergraduate Students*. Malden, MA: Blackwell.

James, V. & McLeod Clark, J. (2007) Benchmarking research development in nursing: Curran's competitive advantage as a framework for excellence. *Journal of Research in Nursing* 12(3): 269–87.

Jinks, A. M. & Green, H. E. (2004) Clinical and academic perspectives on how to develop and enhance nursing research activities. *Journal of Research in Nursing* 9(6): 401–10.

Time management

By the end of this section you will have discovered:

- How to plan your work;
- How to use time effectively.

================= **EXERCISE 9.1** =================

Aim of the exercise: Planning your research project in terms of time.

What to do: You are going to use the process known as 'outlining'. First, jot down on a sheet of paper, the broad stages of your research project, for example:

- planning stage
- searching the literature
- collecting data
- analysing data
- writing up.

Now consider how much time you think you will have available for each broad state and write that time-allowance down next to each heading.

Then take each of these stages in turn and write down sub-tasks that have to be completed in order to complete that stage and time that sub-task, for example:

- Planning stage (two weeks)

    - Identifying area of interest (two days)

    - Choosing research question/problem (two days)

    - Discussion and contract-setting with supervisor (two days)

    - Identifying resources and constraints (two days)

    - Drawing up timetable for the whole of the project (two days)

    - Negotiating access to data collection site (two days).

Notice how quickly your time gets used up. When you have completed each stage, identify to what degree you need to cut back on certain sub-stages. It is useful if you consider your planning under the following three headings:

- What *must* be done

- What *should* be done

- What *could* be done (if time is available)

After you have completed this planning task, draw up a 'master plan' of your research project, showing how aspects of your work will fit into a time scale. Notice that some tasks will run concurrently with others or overlap with others.

Discuss your plan with your supervisor and with your colleagues. Ask them to play 'devil's advocate' and look for problems in your planning. Time spent at this stage is time well spent in that an organized approach will help your project to run smoothly.

Aspects of time management

DO:

- Keep detailed notes as you progress through your project.

- Be disciplined in your approach: if you plan to do something, DO IT!

- Keep your reference cards or computer file up-to-date and make sure that ALL details of the reference are recorded.

- Be systematic in your work.

- Keep in touch with your supervisor.

- Ask lots of questions of people who are more experienced.

DON'T

- Don't leave everything to the last minute: work through your project systematically.

- Don't expect your supervisor to do your project for you.

- Don't expect your supervisor to see you without an appointment: they will have a busy schedule as well.

- Don't expect your library to have all the references you require; plan ahead for books and articles that may take some time to get.

How you manage your time will determine the extent to which you succeed and the quality of your work. A few simple pointers may help to keep you on track:

- Plan your time in a scheduled way and always leave some spare time to deal with the unexpected (which nearly always happens).

- If possible use some diary/calendar software which can be revised when necessary.

- Break up difficult tasks into smaller and more manageable ones wherever possible.

- Try to stick to the allotted times and if your time estimates are poor revise them.

- Have a decent schedule of activities and work in each day and week – challenge yourself.

Robson (2002, p. 54) makes the following points about time management and doing your research project:

Any real world study must obviously take serious note of real world constraints. Your choice of research focus must be realistic in terms of the time and resources that you have available. If you have a maximum of three weeks you can devote to the project, you choose something where you have a good chance of 'getting it out' in that time. Access and co-operation are similarly important, as well as having a good nose for situations where any enquiry is likely to be counter-productive (getting into a sensitive situation involving, say, the siting of a hostel for mentally handicapped adults when your prime aim is to develop community provision is not very sensible if a likely outcome is the stirring up of a hornet's nest).

Budgeting a research project

Most diploma and undergraduate research projects will not require special funding. It is expected that you will work out your proposal so that no 'extra' costs are involved. For example, it will probably be anticipated that you will pay for your own paper for questionnaires, do your own typing or word processing and pay for any local travelling that you have to do. As you move on, however, and do postgraduate or become involved in funded projects, you will have to work out a *budget* for the project. Bear in mind, though, that *all* research projects involve *some* costs and it is worth knowing about how professional researchers budget their programmes.

Here are some examples of the sorts of items that may need to be costed in a larger scale research project. If you have occasion to apply for grants, scholarships or awards, it is likely that you will be asked to prepare a statement of projected costs. Not all funding bodies will ask for all of the following details but read them through and see which ones might apply to your own work.

Personnel

- Salary of research assistant (full or part-time)
- Salary of clerical assistant (full or part-time)
- Training of interviewers
- Computer software training for personnel

Travelling expenses

Travel to interview sites

- Local travel to libraries and appointments
- Travel, fees and accommodation at conferences (national and/or international)

Office equipment

- Computing equipment

- Printers (usually a laser printer)
- Computer software
- Office space
- Telephone rental
- Fax and modem equipment
- Photocopying equipment
- Paper and other stationery
- Cost of instrument/scales

Use of facilities

- Use of library (including searching facilities)
- Use of abstracting services
- Postage

Add-on administrative costs

- Many colleges and universities take a percentage of any research monies that are attracted by their staff. This percentage should be accounted for in any initial budgeting.

Supervision of your research project

A supervisor is the person who oversees your research project. He or she will usually be a lecturer in the department in which you are studying. If you are undertaking a project in your workplace rather than as part of a course of study, then identify a colleague who has undertaken research and ask them if they are prepared to offer you support or if they can recommend someone who could fill the role of supervisor. Supervisors will usually have successfully completed research of their own and may be working on current research projects of their own. They are a valuable resource.

By the end of this section you will have discovered:

- What you can expect of your supervisor;
- What your supervisor can expect of you.

========================= **EXERCISE 9.2** =========================

Aim of the exercise: To explore the role of the supervisor.

What to do: Sit down and write out a list entitled 'What I expect from a supervisor'. You may want to consider such issues as:

- 'She will help me to plan my work'
- 'She will discuss aspects of the methodology'
- 'She will offer constructive criticism of my work', etc.

Now ask your supervisor to undertake a similar exercise. Ask her to write down *two* lists: 'What I can offer as a supervisor' and 'What I expect from you'.

A note about supervision

If you are in the fortunate position of knowing who you would like to supervise your work and already have a good relationship with that person – that is all to the good. However, not everyone can be so lucky. Some people may have to seek out a suitable supervisor and a place of study and this can be a tricky business. A good choice will lead to a productive time whereas a poor choice can lead to wasted time and poor performance. The choice of research supervisor is especially important if you are considering postgraduate studies. Here are some of the key questions you need to think about:

- Are there other students working on similar topics?
- Have I gathered sufficient information about the school or department?
- Who is available to be my supervisor and have they supervised students before successfully?
- What resources for research students are available? (rooms, computers, photocopying, software, library access, etc.)
- What is the research culture like? Do students and staff meet as a group to talk about their work?
- What is the role of the supervisor in this institution? Has the supervisor got time to meet regularly with me? Will he or she provide written feedback?

■ Will my supervisor provide me with a balance between encouraging and supporting me and challenging me to do the best that I can?

■ Which potential supervisors have the most suitable professional and academic background to offer supervision? Do I need to have small group of supervisors who provide input from different perspectives?

The link below provides a detailed example of the range of things that you need to consider at the outset and through the project:

http://www.rsc.qut.edu.au/pdfs/Candidature/Supervisors/tracking_ supervision.pdf

A checklist for achieving good research supervision

The successful completion of a research project is probably one of the most difficult facets of any project. Completing such a project is very much a joint venture involving a research student and a supervisor. Listed below are some questions which can help promote good supervisory practice.

Supervisor

1. What steps are taken to make a good match between a supervisor and the student at a school or department level?

2. Does the supervisor allocate adequate time to meet with the student consistently?

3. Does the supervisor have sufficient time to supervise several students at once?

4. Does the supervisor insist on regular written material throughout the project?

5. Does the supervisor insist on setting aims for the next meeting?

6. Has the supervisor demonstrated how to make systematic records?

7. Does the supervisor help the student to select problems, stimulate and enthuse the student and provide a steady stream of good ideas and guidance?

8. Does the supervisor have expertise in the topic area of the project?

9. Would a supervision team be more suitable to the task and provide methodological expertise coupled with an advanced understanding of the area from a practice perspective?

10. If a team approach is used how often does the team meet with the student?

Student

1. Have you devoted sufficient time into the planning of your project?

2. Have you developed a consistent 'work ethic' that will ensure that the project is completed on time?

3. Have you identified key problem areas?

4. Do you understand the relevant literature?

5. Do you follow up on suggestions offered by more experienced people?

6. Do you keep accurate and systematic records of what you read and what you do?

7. Do you write up your project in small increments as you progress from beginning to end?

8. Do you approach your supervisor when requiring help, giving adequate time for an appointment to be made and, where appropriate, specifying the problem?

9. Do you keep an open mind when receiving feedback on your work?

10. Have you met with your supervisor to review your understanding of the roles and responsibilities of students and supervisors?

SUGGESTED READING

Abidden, N. Z. & West, M. (2007) Effective meeting in graduate student supervision. *Journal of Social Sciences* 3(1): 27–35.

Thompson, D. R., Kirkman, S., Watson, R. & Stewart, S. (2005) Improving research supervision in nursing. *Nurse Education Today* 25: 283–90.

CONCLUSION

In this book we have tried to show you that you can do research. The main theme running through this particular chapter has been the need to be planned and systematic in your approach. While research is not easy, it is easier if you plan it well. Also, the need to be systematic is part of the research process itself: you cannot claim validity for your project if you cannot account for certain aspects of it.

Further, the systematic approach needs to be sustained. As with all things, there are peaks and troughs in any project. The systematic approach will help you to keep going when you are less than enthusiastic about what you are doing. Systematic planning can also point to certain 'maintenance tasks' – filing, checking references and so on – that can help you maintain a sense of impetus.

Note, also, that the efficient planner will think in terms of the 'sub-goals' described above. A sense of achievement will be reinforced by having achieved each of these smaller sub-goals. On the other hand, if you do *not* break down tasks in this way, you may find yourself daunted by the apparent magnitude of the work that is in front of you. In the final chapter, we consider how to write up your work.

10

Writing the Research Report

These are:

- To identify the stages in writing up a research report;

- To consider how to submit a research report to a journal for consideration for publication;

Introduction

All research has to be 'written up'. The reasons for this are fairly clear:

- A research report demonstrates how you have carried out your work and how you reached your conclusions.

- A research report allows you to share your findings with others.

- A research report adds to the body of knowledge in a particular discipline and allows others to critically assess your work and to develop it.

- In human research there is an expectation that you will provide a summary of the findings to participants who wish to have this. This is in keeping with the notion of respectful ethical research.

You may also want to have your research report considered for publication in a nursing magazine or journal. In this way, your work reaches a wider audience.

SUGGESTED READING

This should include the following:

Burnard, P. (2004a) *Writing Skills in Health Care* (2nd edn). Gloucester: Nelson Thornes.

Burnard, P. (2004b) Writing a qualitative research report. *Nurse Education Today* 24: 174–9.

Ritter, R. M. (ed.) (2003) *The Oxford Style Manual.* Oxford: Oxford University Press.

Smyth, T. R. (1996) *Writing in Psychology* (2nd edn). Brisbane: John Wiley & Sons.

Sternberg, R. J. (2003) *The Psychologist's Companion: A Guide to Scientific Writing for Students and Researchers* (4th edn). Cambridge, UK: Cambridge University Press.

Planning your research report

By the end of this section you will have discovered:

- The structure of a research report;
- How to write clearly;
- How to write for publication.

=========== **EXERCISE 10.1** ===========

Aim of the exercise: To explore various ways of structuring a research report.

What to do: Go to the library and study the following research reports. Make notes under the following headings:

- What headings does the writer use to structure the report?
- What differences are there in writing up a qualitative study and a quantitative study?

■ To what degree did illustrations and tables help or hinder your understanding of the research findings?

■ Which journal/s are the most likely to suit your topic?

■ What style of report writing does the journal/s that you might be publishing in use?

■ What skills do you need to develop in order to write in the style that your probable choice of journal/s use?

The studies to review are:

SUGGESTED READING

Burnard, P. and Morrison, P. (2005) Nurses' perceptions of their interpersonal skills: A descriptive study using six category intervention analysis. *Nurse Education Today* 25: 612–17.

Burton, C. R., Fisher, A. & Green, T. L. (2009) The organisational context of nursing care in stroke units: A case study. *International Journal of Nursing Studies* 46(1): 86–95.

Fealy, G., McCarron, M., O'Neill, D., McCallion, P., Clarke, M., Small, V., O'Driscoll, A. & Cullen, A. (2009) Effectiveness of gerontologically informed nursing assessment and referral interventions for older persons attending the emergency department: Systematic review. *Journal of Advanced Nursing* 65(5): 934–45.

Gilmour, J. A., Scott, S. D. & Huntington, N. (2007) Nurses and Internet health information: A questionnaire survey. *Journal of Advanced Nursing* 61(1): 19–28.

Holmes, S. (2009) Methodological and ethical considerations in designing an Internet study of quality of life: A discussion paper. *International Journal of Nursing Studies* 46(3): 394–405.

Huntington, A., Gilmour, J., Schluter, P., Tuckett, A., Bogossian, F. & Turner, C. (2009) The Internet as a research site: Establishment of a web-based longitudinal study of the nursing and midwifery workforce in three countries. *Journal of Advanced Nursing* 65(6): 1309–17.

Scott, S.D., Gilmour, J. & Fielden, J. (2008) Nursing students and Internet health information. *Nurse Education Today* 28(8): 993–1001.

Yu, J. & Kirk, M. (2008) Measurement of empathy in nursing research: Systematic review. *Journal of Advanced Nursing* 64(5): 440–54.

There is no 'right way' to structure a research report. However, certain headings and sub-headings occur in many studies. If you have followed a logical sequence of events in doing your research, that sequence should guide you to the structuring of your report. Headings that you may want to consider are as follows:

1. Title

2. Summary

3. Precise statement of the scope and aims of the study

4. Rationale for the study

5. Review of the literature

6. Methods

7. Results/Findings

8. Discussion

9. Conclusions and recommendations

10. References

11. Appendices.

Writing your report

By the end of this section you will have discovered:

- How to write clearly;
- The materials needed for a write-up;
- How to present your write-up.

=========== **EXERCISE 10.2** ===========

Aim of the exercise: To explore approaches to writing a research report.

What to do: Go to a college or university library and ask to see copies of theses submitted for research degrees (MSc, MPhil, PhD). Select a small range of these to peruse and try to choose studies from different fields and subject areas. Remember too that people who have successfully supervised honours, masters and PhD projects will have copies of these. Alternatively you could look through some of the following thesis databases and find some PhD studies that interest you:

http://adt.caul.edu.au/
http://www.theses.com/

http://www.ndltd.org/
http://dspace.mit.edu/
http://etext.virginia.edu/ETD/
http://www.collectionscanada.gc.ca/thesescanada/

As you look through these dissertations and theses, make notes on the following:

■ How are the words laid out on the page: what line-spacing has been used?

■ What size margins have been used?

■ Are the pages numbered?

■ Is there a table of contents?

■ Have appendices been used for additional material?

■ Is the report written on both sides of the page or only on one?

■ Are headings used and, if so, how?

■ How is the report bound?

■ How is the list of references presented?

Consider, also, whether there are particular rules about the presentation of your research project that are peculiar to your college or school. Usually there are written details of how to prepare a research report for your organization.

Bear in mind that the reports we have asked you to look at are reports submitted for higher degrees. We do not anticipate that you will necessarily be writing in this way. The reports do, however, offer good examples of a standard approach and layout for presenting a written report of a research project.

Writing clearly

■ Use short sentences.

■ Do not use long words when simpler ones would do.

■ Keep jargon and technical terms to a minimum.

■ Do not use long paragraphs. If you plan your writing, you can divide up what you have to say into manageable 'chunks'.

■ Use headings to guide the reader.

■ Remember *who* you are writing for: the audience for your writing may dictate the style.

- Edit your work frequently. Cut out all unnecessary words and phrases. Avoid 'padding'.

- Be prepared to make several drafts of your report.

- Show your work (a) to your supervisor, for comments and (b) to an 'outsider', who has nothing to do with the field. Listen to the latter's comments carefully.

If necessary, consult a style manual to help you to present your findings and to learn to use the appropriate style for writing research reports such as:

SUGGESTED READING

Turabian, K. (2007) *A Manual for Writers of Research Papers, Theses, and Dissertations: Chicago Style for Students and Researchers* (7th edn). Chicago: The University of Chicago Press (particularly pp. 62–132).

Consider reading the following which will also help to write well:

Peat, J., Elliot, E., Baur, L. & Keena, V. (2002) *Scientific Writing: Easy When You Know How*. London: BMJ Books (particularly pp. 1–44 and 188–272).

Silvia, P. J. (2007) *How to Write a Lot. A Practical Guide to Productive Academic Writing*. Washington, DC: American Psychological Association (skim the whole book and then reread in detail those chapters that are particularly useful to you).

Perrin, R. (2009) *Pocket Guide to APA Style* (3rd edn). Boston: Wadsworth, pp. 1–58.

Working with a computer

Many people, nowadays, write directly to a computer screen, using a word processing package. This is a particularly economical way of using your time and is much better than writing longhand and then transferring your work to the computer. Here are some points about the use of a word processor and writing a research report:

- Get to know your computer well. Most people use personal computers (PC) and many others use Apple computers. It is a personal choice as most of the files people work on are almost completely interchangeable these days. In preparing this book two of us used a PC and the other an iMac.

■ Try to learn *all* of the functions of your word processor. Many people use word processors as glorified typewriters but this is to miss the point. Used fully, a word processor can help you to check your spelling and grammar, count your words, enable you to transfer data from one part of a document to another, compile an index for your report, produce a table of contents, and enable you to produce a professional-looking document.

■ Divide your report up into small sections and open up a new file for each section. Many word processors have a function that allows you to quickly and easily draw together a number of related files into a 'master-file' that allows you to view the whole of your document as one piece of work.

■ Save your work regularly and make back-ups of your work to an external hard disk or USB flash drive. On the other hand, also make full use of your hard disk. Some people get into the odd habit of working from USB flash drives and using the hard disk only for storing programs. This, again, is to miss the point of working with computers. A hard disk is much faster.

■ Do not make *lots* of 'hard copies' of your work (a hard copy is a printed one). On the other hand, make one such copy just before you print out your *final* report and edit it. It is often easy to miss minor errors when you are reading text on the computer monitor. You should get someone else to proofread your final report before printing off the final copies for binding.

■ Get to know the local 'computer expert'. Do not panic if things go wrong. Stop what you are doing and call the expert. You can often *undelete* files that you think you have lost but *only* if you do not reuse the computer after you have made a major error.

■ Find out what computing facilities are available in your college and make full use of them. Apply to go on software training courses if they are available. Most universities will run sessions on using the major programs they have adopted across the campus including word processing, presentation software and bibliographic management such as EndNote®. On the other hand, do not feel that you have to learn to *program* with a computer. These days, not many users have to develop programming skills but *all* have to learn to use the software that is available.

Writing for publication

By the end of this section you will have discovered:

- How to prepare your work for publication;
- How to acquire guidelines for publication.

Opportunities for publication

Your report may be considered for publication by a number of organizations. Some opportunities for publishing your work include:

- As a journal article
- As a 'short report' in a journal of abstracts
- As a chapter in a book
- As a book
- As a monograph published by your college, school or university department
- As a published conference paper
- As a local report in your organization.

Reasons for publishing research reports

Strauss and Corbin, in a discussion about writing and publishing parts of theses and monographs, offer the following points about publishing research:

1. ... researchers may decide to publish papers even relatively early during the research process. They may do this for different reasons. For instance, to present preliminary findings, or to satisfy or impress sponsors, or because they have interesting materials bearing on side issues that can easily be written up now but might not get written at a later more hectic time.

2. Sometimes researchers write papers because they feel either obligated to publish on a given topic or because they are pressured to do so. Of course this motivation will also affect what and how a researcher writes.

3. Researchers may also be invited to contribute papers to special issues of journals or edited volumes, because they are known to be researching in given areas. They may also be urged or tempted to convert verbal presentations into papers, because listeners have responded well to them.

4. Another condition that can affect the writing of a paper is the existence of a deadline for getting the finished product to an editor. For some researchers this can act as a stimulus, while others of course are daunted by any deadline.

5. The number of pages allowed by the editor also affects whether a paper will be written – at least for this particular publication – and what will be written and how.

6. Unless invited by an editor, there is the important decision to be made about which particular journal should be elected as a potential outlet for a given paper. Journals and papers have to be matched, otherwise time is wasted in its rejection, or worse yet the paper is accepted but for an inappropriate or insufficiently appreciative audience.

(Strauss and Corbin 1998)

Reporting your findings to respondents and others

There are various ways that others can learn of your research. Some methods of disseminating your findings include:

- Discussion groups in the school of nursing or where you are currently working;

- Submitting an abstract to a conference;

- Inviting respondents to a study day;

- Through a local research interest group;

- Local publications within the school, college or university.

======================= **EXERCISE 10.3** =======================

Aim of the exercise: To explore research reports that have been published.

What to do: Obtain a small sample of research reports (books and journals) from the library. Read them and make notes under the following headings:

- Was the report interesting?

- Was the report relevant: did it have implications for practice or for further research?

- Did the writer's style keep your attention or was it difficult to finish reading the paper or book?

- Would you have read it by choice?

■ Would it have wide appeal?

Now study the following books on writing for publication:

SUGGESTED READING

Cargill, M. & O'Connor, P. (2009) *Writing Scientific Research Articles: Strategies and Steps.* Oxford: Wiley Blackwell.

Belcher, W. (2009) *Writing Your Journal Article in 12 Weeks: A Guide to Academic Publishing Success.* Thousand Oaks: Sage.

Sternberg, R. J. (2003) *The Psychologist's Companion: A Guide to Scientific Writing for Students and Researchers* (4th edn). Cambridge, UK: Cambridge University Press.

Discuss your findings with your colleagues and draw out the ingredients of a good published report. Remember that, from the publisher's point of view, the main question is 'Will this article or book *sell?*' Note that this raises different evaluation criteria from those that apply to evaluating research reports that are not for publication. A written report may be excellent but it will not get published if it does not help to sell the book or journal. But... keep trying! The value to yourself and others of having a report published is worth the effort.

Submitting work for consideration for publication

Getting your report published may be an important aspect of the sharing and development of knowledge. While you may have to wait a while before you see your work published, and there can be no guarantee that your work will be accepted, the following guidelines may help to speed up the process:

■ Approach one journal with the *idea* of your report. This allows you and the publisher to know whether there is a likelihood of acceptance for publication.

■ Only submit to one journal at a time. It is also illegal to publish the same piece of work in two journals, without permission from the first publisher.

■ Get a copy of their 'Advice to Authors' from the internet. Follow the guidelines to the letter. Sometimes this information is contained inside the back page of the journal itself.

- Most journals now use on-line submission but if you are sending a hard copy prepare only blemish-free copies. A scruffy manuscript is unlikely to impress editors.

- Be prepared for a journal to reject your work. Some will write back with details of how your work could be modified. Others will not. If you do get advice on how to revise your work, follow that advice carefully. The editor always knows best.

- Keep a copy of anything you submit for publication and note the date on which you send work off to journals.

CONCLUSION

You have now completed your research. Now you can consider your next move: will you do more research, further study...another course? Your work has stopped for the moment but, if you are to continue your research journey, you need to consider the next step. We hope that you have enjoyed working through this book and through the process of research. Good luck!

References

Abidden, N. Z. & West, M. (2007) Effective meeting in graduate student supervision. *Journal of Social Sciences* 3(1): 27–35.

Alreck, P. L. & Settle, R. B. (2004) *The Survey Research Handbook* (3rd edn). Columbus, OH: McGraw-Hill.

Anthonak, R. F. and Livneh, H. (1988) *The Measurement of Attitudes Towards People with Disabilities: Methods, Psychometrics and Scales.* Springfield, Illinois: Charles C. Thomas.

Anthony, S. & Jack, S. (2009) Qualitative case study methodology in nursing research: An integrative review. *Journal of Advanced Nursing* 65(6): 1171–81.

Aranda, S., Schofield, P., Weih, L., Milne, D., Yates, P. & Faulkner, R. (2006) Meeting the support and information needs of women with advanced breast cancer: A randomised controlled trial. *The British Journal of Cancer* 95(6): 667.

Barker, C. & Pistrang, N. (2005) Quality criteria under methodological pluralism: Implications for conducting and evaluating research. *American Journal of Community Psychology* 35: 201–12.

Barredo, RDV & Dudley, T. J. (2008) A descriptive study of losses associated with permanent long-term care placement. *Journal of Geriatric Physical Therapy* 31(3): 87–92.

Beecroft, C., Rees, A. & Booth, A. (2009) Finding the evidence. In K. Gerrish & A. Lacey (eds) *The Research Process in Nursing.* Oxford: Blackwell Publishing, pp. 95–7.

Belcher, W. (2009) *Writing Your Journal Article in 12 weeks: A Guide to Academic Publishing Success.* Thousand Oaks: Sage.

Bell, J. (2005) *Doing Your Research Project: A Guide for First-time Researchers in Education and Social Science* (4th edn). Milton Keynes: Open University Press.

Berg, B. L. (2008) *Qualitative Research Methods for the Social Sciences* (7th edn). Boston, MA: Allyn & Bacon.

Bernardo, L. M., Matthews, J. T., Kaufmann, J. A. & Yang, K. (2008) Promoting critical appraisal of the research literature: A workshop for school nurses. *The Journal of Continuing Education in Nursing* 39(10): 461–7.

Borbasi, S., Jackson, D. & Langford, R. (2008) *Navigating the Maze of Nursing Research* (2nd edn). Marrackville: Elsevier.

Boswell, C. & Cannon, S. (2007) *Introduction to Nursing Research: Incorporating Evidence-Based Practice.* Sudbury, MA: Jones and Bartlett.

Bowling, A. (2001) *Measuring Disease. A Review of Disease Specific Quality of Life Measurement Scales* (2nd edn). Buckingham: Open University Press/McGraw-Hill.

Bowling, A. (2004) *Measuring Health: A Review of Quality of Life Measurement Scales* (3rd edn). Milton Keynes: Open University Press.

Bradburn, N. M., Sudman, S. & Wansink, B. (2004) *Asking Questions: The Definitive to Questionnaire Design for Market Research, Political Polls, and Social and Health Questionnaires.* San Francisco: Jossey Bass.

Burnard, P. (2004a) *Writing Skills in Health Care* (2nd edn). Gloucester: Nelson Thornes.

Burnard, P. (2004b) Writing a qualitative research report. *Nurse Education Today* 24: 174–9.

Burnard, P. and Morrison, P. (2005) Nurses' perceptions of their interpersonal skills: A descriptive study using six category intervention analysis. *Nurse Education Today* 25: 612–17.

Burton, C. R., Fisher, A. & Green, T. L. (2009) The organisational context of nursing care in stroke units: A case study. *International Journal of Nursing Studies* 46(1): 86–95.

Cargill, M. & O'Connor, P. (2009) *Writing Scientific Research Articles: Strategies and Steps.* Oxford: Wiley Blackwell.

Coolican, H. (2009) *Research Methods and Statistics in Psychology* (5th edn). London: Hodder Arnold.

Coxon, A. P. M. (1999) *Sorting Data: Collection and Analysis.* London: Sage Publication.

Coyne, I. T. (1997) Sampling in qualitative research. Purposeful and theoretical sampling; merging or clear boundaries? *Journal of Advanced Nursing* 26: 623–30.

Crang, M. & Cook, I. (2007) *Doing Ethnographies.* London: Sage.

Creswell, J. (2007) *Qualitative Inquiry & Research Design: Choosing Among Five Approaches* (2nd edn). California: Sage Publications, pp. 202–13.

Creswell, J. & Plano-Clark, V. (2011) *Designing and Conducting Mixed Methods Research.* California: Sage, pp. 1–18.

Creswell, J. W. (2009) *Research Design: Qualitative, Quantitative, and Mixed Methods Approaches* (3rd edn). London: Sage.

Davies, M. B. (2007) *Doing a Successful Research Project: Using Qualitative or Quantitative Methods.* Basingstoke: Palgrave Macmillan.

Day, J., Higgins, I. & Koch, T. (2009) The process of practice redesign in delirium care for hospitalised older people: A participatory action research study. *International Journal of Nursing Studies* 46(1):13–22.

de Bono, E. (1990) *Lateral Thinking: A Textbook of Creativity.* Harmondsworth: Penguin.

Doney, R. M. & Packer, T. L. (2008) Measuring changes in activity participation of older Australians: Validation of the Activity Card Sort-Australia. *Australian Journal of Ageing* 27(1): 33–7.

Edvardsson, D. (2009) Balancing between being a person and being a patient – a qualitative study of wearing patient clothing. *International Journal of Nursing Studies* 46: 4–11.

Edwards, H., Courtney, M., Finlayson, K., Shuter, P. & Lindsay, E. (2009) A randomized controlled trial of a community nursing intervention: Improved quality of life and healing for clients with chronic leg ulcers. *Journal of Clinical Nursing* 18(11): 1541–9.

Fealy, G., McCarron, M., O'Neill, D., McCallion, P., Clarke, M., Small, V., O'Driscoll, A. & Cullen, A. (2009) Effectiveness of gerontologically informed nursing assessment and referral interventions for older persons attending the emergency department: Systematic review. *Journal of Advanced Nursing* 65(5): 934–45.

Flanagan, J. C. (1954) The critical incident technique. *Psychological Bulletin* 51(4): 327–58.

Flick, U. (2007) *Designing Qualitative Research.* London: Sage.

Fransella, F. (ed.) (2005) *The Essential Practitioner's Handbook of Personal Construct Psychology.* Chichester: Wiley.

Fransella, F., Bell, R. & Bannister, D. (2003) *A Manual for Repertory Grid Technique* (2nd edn). Chichester: Wiley.

Fraser, L. & Lawley, M. (2000) *Questionnaire Design & Administration: A Practical Guide.* Brisbane, Australia: John Wiley & Sons.

Gerrish, K. & Lacey, A. (eds) (2006) *The Research Process in Nursing* (5th edn). Oxford: Blackwell Publishing.

Gill, P. & Burnard, P. (2008) The student-supervisor relationship in the PhD/Doctoral process. *British Journal of Nursing* 17(10): 668–71.

Gilmour, J. A. Scott, S. D. & Huntington, N. (2007) Nurses and Internet health information: A questionnaire survey. *Journal of Advanced Nursing* 61(1): 19–28.

Godshall, M. (2010) *Fast Facts for Evidence Based Practice: Implementing EBP in a Nutshell.* New York: Springer Publishers.

Golafshani, N. (2003) Understanding reliability and validity in qualitative research. *The Qualitative Report* 8(4): 597–607.

Goldsmith, L., Skirton, H. & Webb, C. (2008) Informed consent to healthcare interventions in people with learning disabilities – an integrative review. *Journal of Advanced Nursing* 64(6): 549–63.

Goodman, C. & Evans, C. (2006) Using focus groups. In K. Gerrish & A. Lacey (eds) *The Research Process in Nursing.* Oxford: Blackwell Publishing.

Gould, D. (2008) Undertaking a research project: Guidance for nursing students. *Nursing Standard* 22(50): 48–54.

Graneheim, U. H. & Lundman, B. (2004) Qualitative content analysis in nursing research: Concepts, procedures and measures to achieve trustworthiness. *Nurse Education Today* 24(2): 105–12.

Hammersley, M. (1992) *What's Wrong with Ethnography?* London: Routledge.

Hardy, D. J., O'Brien, A. P., Gaskin, C. J., O'Brien, A. J., Morrison-Ngatai, E., Skews, G., Ryan, T. & McNulty, N. (2004) Practical application of the Delphi Technique in a bicultural mental health nursing study in New Zealand. *Journal of Advanced Nursing* 46(1): 95–109.

Hart, M. (2007) Birthing a research project: Sampling. *International Journal of Childbirth Education* 22(2): 31–4.

Hewitt, J. (2007) Ethical consideration of researcher-researched relationships in qualitative interviewing. *Qualitative Health Research* 17(8): 1149–59.

Higginbottom, G. (2005) Ethical footprints: Finding a way through the research process. *Nurse Researcher* 13(2): 4–6.

Holmes, S. (2009) Methodological and ethical considerations in designing an Internet study of quality of life: A discussion paper. *International Journal of Nursing Studies* 46(3): 394–405.

Huntington, A., Gilmour, J., Schluter, P., Tuckett, A., Bogossian, F. & Turner, C. (2009) The Internet as a research site: Establishment of a web-based longitudinal study of the nursing and midwifery workforce in three countries. *Journal of Advanced Nursing* 65(6): 1309–17.

James, V. & McLeod Clark, J. (2007) Benchmarking research development in nursing: Curran's competitive advantage as a framework for excellence. *Journal of Research in Nursing* 12(3): 269–87.

Jankowicz, A. D. (2003) *The Easy Guide to Repertory Grids*. Chichester: Wiley, pp. 8–31.

Jinks, A. M. & Green, H. E. (2004) Clinical and academic perspectives on how to develop and enhance nursing research activities. *Journal of Research in Nursing* 9(6): 401–10.

Keatinge, D. (2002) Versatility and flexibility: Attributes of the critical incident technique in nursing research. *Nursing & Health Sciences* 4(1–2): 33–9.

Keeney, S. Hasson, F. & McKenna, H. (2006) Consulting the oracle: Ten lessons from using the Delphi technique in nursing research. *Journal of Advanced Nursing* 53(2): 205–12.

Kelly, G. A. (1955) *The Psychology of Personal Constructs*, 2 vols. New York: Norton.

Kemppainen, J. K. (2001) The critical incident technique and nursing care quality research. *Journal of Advanced Nursing* 32(5): 1264–71.

Kitson, A. (2002) Recognising relationships: Reflections on evidence-based practice. *Nursing Inquiry* 9(3): 179–86.

Krosnic, J. & Presser, S. (2010) Questions and questionnaire design. In J. Wright & Marsden (eds) *Handbook of Survey Research* (2nd edn). San Diego, CA: Elsevier, pp. 263–315.

Kvale, S. & Brinkman, S. (2009) *Interviews: Learning the Craft of Qualitative Research Interviewing* (2nd edn). London: Sage.

Lacey, A. (2006) The research process. In K. Gerrish & A. Lacey (eds) *The Research Process in Nursing* (5th edn). Oxford: Blackwell Publishing.

Leedy, P. D. & Ormrod, J. E. (2001) *Practical Research: Planning and Design* (7th edn). New Jersey: Merrill Prentice Hall.

Levett-Jones, T., Lathlean, J., Higgins, I. & McMillan, M. (2008/9) The duration of clinical placements: A key influence on nursing students' experience of belongingness. *Australian Journal of Advanced Nursing* 26(2): 8–16.

Lewin, K. (1946) Action research and minority problems. *Journal of Social Issues* 2: 34–46.

Linstone, H. & Turoff, M. (1975) http://is.njit.edu/pubs/delphibook/.

Lumsden, J. (2007) Online questionnaire design. In R. Reynolds & R. Woods (eds) *Handbook of Research on Electronic Survey Measurement*. London: Idea Group Reference, pp. 44–64.

Lyneham, J. Parkinson, C. & Denholm, C. (2008) Intuition in emergency nursing: A phenomenological study. *International Journal of Nursing Practice* 14: 101–8.

Macnee, C. L. & McCabe, S. (2008) *Understanding Nursing Research: Reading and Using Research in Evidence-Based Practice* (2nd edn). Philadelphia: Lippincott, Williams & Wilkins.

Mantzoukas, S. (2009) The research evidence published in high impact nursing journals between 2000–2006: A quantitative content analysis. *International Journal of Nursing Studies* 46(4): 479–89.

Marshall, M., Carter, B., Rose, K. & Brotherton, A. (2009) Living with type 1 diabetes: Perspectives of children and their parents. *Journal of Clinical Nursing* 18(12): 1703–10.

May, T. (1993) *Social Research: Issues, Method and Process*. Milton Keynes: Open University.

McBrien, B. (2008) Evidence-based care: Enhancing the rigour of a qualitative study. *British Journal of Nursing* 17(20): 286–9.

McDowell, I. & Newell, C. (1996) *Measuring Health. A Guide to Rating Scales and Questionnaires* (2nd edn). New York: Oxford University Press.

Meadows, K. A. (2003) So you want to do research? 5: Questionnaire design. *British Journal of Community Nursing* 8(12): 562–70.

Miller, D. C. (2002) *Handbook of Research Design and Social Measurement* (6th edn). Newbury Park: Sage.

Minichiello, V., Sullivan, G., Greenwood, K. & Axford, R. (eds) (2004) *Handbook for Research Methods for Nursing and Health Sciences*. Frenchs Forest, NSW: Prentice-Hall.

Mitchell, T. & Caroll, J. (2008) Academic and research misconduct in the PhD: Issues for students and supervisors. *Nurse Education Today* 28(2): 218–26.

Narayanasamy, A., Clissett, P., Parumal, L., Thompson, D., Annasamy, S. & Edge, R. (2004) Responses to the spiritual needs of older people. *Journal of Advanced Nursing* 48(1): 6–16.

Neuendorf, K. (2002) *The Content Analysis Guidebook*. California: Sage Publications.

Neufeld, A., Harrison, M. J., Rempel, G. R., Larocque, S., Dublin, S., Stewart, M., Hughes, K. (2004) Practical issues in using a card sort in a study of non-support and family care-giving. *Qualitative Health Research* 14: 1418–28.

Newell, R. & Burnard, P. (2010a) *Research for Evidence-Based Practice* (2nd edn). Oxford: Blackwell.

Newell, R. & Burnard, P. (2010b) *Vital Notes for Nurses: Research for Evidence-Based Practice* (2nd edn). Oxford, Blackwell Publishing.

Nkowane, A. M. & Saxena, S. (2004) Opportunities for an improved role for nurses in psychoactive use: Review of the literature. *International Journal of Nursing Practice* 10: 102–10.

Olin, J. T. & Keatinge, C. (1998) *Rapid Psychological Assessment*. New York: Wiley.

Oppenheim, A. N. (1992) *Questionnaire Design, Interviewing and Attitude Measurement* (2nd edn). London: Pinter.

Peat, J., Elliot, E., Baur, L. & Keena, V. (2002) *Scientific Writing: Easy When You Know How*. London: BMJ Books, (particularly pp. 1–44 and 188–272).

Perrin, R. (2009) *Pocket Guide to APA Style* (3rd edn). Boston: Wadsworth, pp. 1–58.

Pivik, J., Rode, E. & Ward, C. (2004) A consumer involvement model for health technology assessment in Canada. *Health Policy* 69(2): 253–68.

Polit, D. & Beck, C. (2010) *Essentials of Nursing Research: Appraising Evidence for Nursing Practice*. Philadelphia: Lippincott Williams & Wilkins.

Powell, C. (2003) The Delphi technique: Myths and realities. *Journal of Advanced Nursing* 41(4): 376–82.

Price, B. (2002) Laddered questions and qualitative data research interviews. *Journal of Advanced Nursing* 37: 273–81.

Punch, K. (2005) *Introduction to Social Research: Quantitative and Qualitative Approaches* (2nd edn). London: Sage Publishing.

Ralley, C., Allott, R., Hare, D.J., Wittkowski, A. (2009) The use of the repertory grid technique to examine staff beliefs about clients with dual diagnosis. *Clinical Psychology & Psychotherapy* 16(2): 148–58.

Reeve, J., James, F. & McNeill, R. (2009) Providing psychosocial and physical rehabilitation advice for patients with burns. *Journal of Advanced Nursing* 65(5): 1039–43.

Rejeh, N., Ahmadi, F., Mohammadi, E., Kazemnejad, A. & Anoosheh, M. (2009) Nurses' experiences and perceptions of influencing barriers to postoperative pain management. *Scandinavian Journal of Caring Sciences* 23(2): 274–81.

Reynolds, T., Russell, L., Deeth, M., Jones, H. & Birchall, L. (2004) A randomised controlled trial comparing Drawtex with standard dressings for exuding wounds. *Journal of Wound Care* 13(2): 71–4.

Ritter, R. M. (ed.) (2003) *The Oxford Style Manual*. Oxford: Oxford University Press.

Robinson, A., Andrews-Hall, S., Cubit, K., Fassett, M., Venter, L., Menzies, B. & Jongeling, L. (2008) Attracting students to aged care: The impact of a supportive orientation. *Nurse Education Today* 28(3): 354–62.

Robinson, J. P., Shaver, P. R. & Wrightman, L. S. (eds) (1991) *Measures of Personality and Social Psychological Attitudes*. San Diego, CA: Academic Press.

Robson, C. (2002) *Real World Research: A Resource for Social Scientists and Practitioner-Researchers* (2nd edn). Oxford: Blackwell.

Robson, C. (2007) *How to Do a Research Project: A Guide for Undergraduate Students*. Oxford: Blackwell Publishing.

Rubin, H. J. & Rubin, I. S. (2005) *Qualitative Interviewing: The Art of Hearing Data* (2nd edn). Thousand Oaks, CA: Sage.

Salkind, N. (2007) *Statistics for People Who (Think They) Hate Statistics* (2nd edn). London: Sage.

Schluter, J., Seaton, P. & Chaboyer, W. (2008) Critical incident technique: A user's guide for nursing researchers. *Journal of Advanced Nursing* 61(1): 107–14.

Scott, S. D., Gilmour, J. & Fielden, J. (2008) Nursing students and Internet health information. *Nurse Education Today* 28(8): 993–1001.

Sheu, S., Wei, I., Chen, C. Yu, S. & Tang, F. (2009) Using snowball sampling method with nurses to understand medication and administration errors. *Journal of Clinical Nursing* 18(4): 559–69.

Shields, L. (2008) Sampling in quantitative research. *Paediatric Nursing* 20(5): 37.

Silvia, P. J. (2007) *How to Write a Lot. A Practical Guide to Productive Academic Writing*. Washington, DC: American Psychological Association.

Smith, K. (2008) Building upon existing evidence to shape future research endeavors. *American Journal of Health System Pharmacy* 65: 1767–74.

Smyth, T. R. (1996) *Writing in Psychology* (2nd edn). Brisbane: John Wiley & Sons.

Sommer, B. & Sommer, R. (2002) *A Practical Guide to Behavioural Research: Tools and Techniques* (5th edn). Oxford: Oxford University Press.

Spencer, D. (2009) *Card Sorting: Designing Usable Categories*. Brooklyn, NY: Rosenfeld Media.

Stein, C. H. & Mankowski, E. S. (2004) Asking, witnessing, interpreting, knowing: Conducting qualitative research in community psychology. *American Journal of Community Psychology* 33: 21–35.

Stephenson, W. (1953) *The Study of Behaviour: Q-Technique and its Methodology*. Chicago: University of Chicago Press.

Sternberg, R. J. (2003) *The Psychologist's Companion: A Guide to Scientific Writing for Students and Researchers* (4th edn). Cambridge, UK: Cambridge University Press.

Strauss, A. & Corbin, J. (1998) *Basics of Qualitative Research Techniques and Procedures for Developing Grounded Theory* (2nd edn). London: Sage.

Tansella, M. & Thornicroft, G. (eds) (2001) *Mental Health Outcome Measures* (2nd edn). London: Gaskell.

Taylor, J., Lauder, W., Moy, M. & Collett, J. (2009) Practitioner assessments of 'good enough' preventing: Factorial survey. *Journal of Clinical Nursing* 18(8): 1180–9.

Taylor, S. & Bogdan, R. (1984) *Introduction to Qualitative Research Methods: The Search for Meaning*. New York: Wiley.

Thompson, D. R., Kirkman, S., Watson, R. & Stewart, S. (2005) Improving research supervision in nursing. *Nurse Education Today* 25: 283–90.

Turabian, K. (2007) *A Manual for Writers of Research Papers, Theses, and Dissertations: Chicago Style for Students and Researchers* (7th edn). Chicago: The University of Chicago Press.

Usher, K., Baker, J. A., Holmes, C. & Stocks, B. (2009) Clinical decision-making for 'as needed' medications in mental health care. *Journal of Advanced Nursing* 65(5): 981–91.

Vernon, W. (2009) The Delphi technique: A review. *International Journal of Therapy and Rehabilitation* 16(2): 69–76.

Watkins, M., Jones, R., Lindsey, L. & Sheaff, R. (2008) The clinical content of NHS trust board meetings: An initial exploration. *Journal of Nursing Management* 16(6): 707–15.

Watson, H. & White, R. (2006) Using observation. In K. Gerrish & A. Lacey (eds) *The Research Process in Nursing*. Oxford: Blackwell Publishing, pp. 383–98.

Winsett, R. P. & Cashion, A. K. (2007) The nursing research process. *Nephrology Nursing Journal* 34(6): 635–43.

Yu, J. & Kirk, M. (2008) Measurement of empathy in nursing research: Systematic review. *Journal of Advanced Nursing* 64(5): 440–54.

Zambas, S. (2010) Purpose of the systematic physical assessment in everyday practice: Critique of the 'Sacred Cow'. *Journal of Nursing Education* 49(6): 305–9.

Zilembo, M. & Monterosso, L. (2008) Nursing students' perceptions of desirable leadership qualities in nurse preceptors: A descriptive survey. *Contemporary Nurse* 27(2): 194–206.

Index